FOR RIDERS OF ALL LEVELS AND DISCIPLINES

Ride in Balance

Expand Your Riding Skills with
Body Awareness and Pilates Exercises

BETH GLOSTEN, MD

RiderPilates® LLC

Michal
Ride in balance & ride
in good health, for years!

Beth

Copyright © 2011 by Beth Glosten

ISBN: 978-0-615-48289-7
Library of Congress Control Number: 2011906822

Printed in the United States of America

Editor: Karen Parkin
Design: Soundview Design Studio
Illustrations: Sandy Johnson
Exercise photographs: Audrey Guidi
Equestrian photographs: Carolynn Bunch Photography (unless otherwise noted)

Front cover photo credits:
Beth on Bluette: Poulsen Photography
Beth with Donner Girl: John Forsen
Beth on ball: Audrey Guidi

www.riderpilates.com

This book is for passionate riders of all
skill levels and disciplines who take seriously
their responsibilities as participants in the
horse-rider team and seek to develop their
riding skills despite struggles with injuries
and training setbacks.

Contents

Exercises

Chapter 1: Keep Mentally Focused

Chapter 2: Maintain Proper Posture

Chapter 3: Control Your Body: Legs

Chapter 4: Control Your Body: Arms

Chapter 5: Understand How Your Horse Moves

Introduction

I am a dressage rider, and for me, like many others, this is no casual pursuit. With some great equine partners, I've trained and competed in dressage from the elementary Training Level up to the advanced Grand Prix, and earned my United States Dressage Federation (USDF) bronze, silver, and gold medals. But along the way I've hit some bumps, including injuries that ultimately led me to examine rider balance and function, develop a Pilates-based exercise program called RiderPilates, and devise the Rider Checklist to help riders use their bodies on horseback in a logical and healthy way.

This didn't happen overnight.

My Story

In 1997 I found myself burnt out and troubled with my job as an academic anesthesiologist and in significant pain from a herniated lumbar disk in my back that required surgery. The pain of the injury jolted my life into acute focus and screamed at me, "You only go around once!" I took the voice seriously and asked my department chair for a leave of absence. I never went back.

Out of the structure of academic medicine and adrift without a schedule, I was bouncing off the walls. After a few months I put on my scientific method hat and researched what I should do for the next phase of my life.

During this time I pursued my physical well-being. I was determined to avoid more back problems, so I religiously performed my physical therapy exercises, read books on the pathophysiology of my back condition and spine mechanics, and sought a logical approach to life and to riding to minimize further degeneration of my body. Fitness was clearly a part of the program. I vowed to do everything possible to continue riding.

By chance, while skimming a local equestrian newspaper, I came across an article about rider fitness. The author taught Pilates, an exercise system that I'd heard of but had never tried. I was intrigued that this instructor knew about horseback riding, so I signed up for some classes.

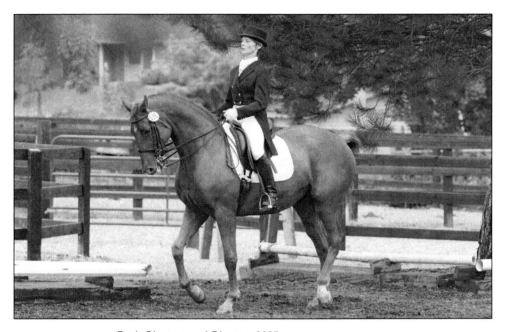

Beth Glosten and Bluette, 2005 (Amber Palmer Photography).

The Pilates instructor was patient and keen. She quickly pointed out postural and movement habits that, in hindsight, likely contributed to my degenerative back problem. "Move just at your hip joint while doing the leg circles, keep your spine stable," she'd say as I struggled with this seemingly simple task. Until I tried Pilates, I had approached my exercises with a "check the box" attitude. I didn't pay attention to *how* I did each exercise. I just did it.

Pilates taught me more than healthy movement. I was confronted with a system that challenged my paradigm that "all problems are solved by working harder." This approach is too easy; life is not so simple. While hard work may be necessary, it is not enough. Most problems require working *smarter*, with discipline and patience that allow time to learn. I realized that it wasn't just muscle strength that I needed to keep my body healthy. I also needed precision and attention to detail. I needed to improve my awareness. And I needed to be patient. Sounds just like dressage, right?

My Pilates sessions often drained me both mentally and physically. But, I found that my best rides were those in the afternoon following a Pilates session. During these rides I had better balance and command over my body. I was able to move with my horse, rather than against him. "What is going on here?" I wondered. I was stunned that dramatic changes in the function of my body could come following a Pilates workout and be translated to improved riding that same day. I hypothesized that Pilates sessions, by focusing on posture, balance, and flexibility, organized my body and my body awareness so that my riding skills immediately improved. I sought more details.

I spent hours analyzing my own riding and that of others, both proficient and not. I began to see how many riders lacked some basic (but *not* easy) skills of core balance and shoulder and leg muscle suppleness. I sought common ground between my growing understanding of healthy body and spine mechanics and what made great riders great. My conclusion? They are one and the same: A great rider's grace, ease, and beauty come from balance and efficient use of the body, and follow healthy principles of proper posture and spine alignment, effective postural support, and control of movement in the entire body. Through Pilates I learned these skills—and the more I learned, the more I wanted to share these ideas.

A great rider's grace, ease, and beauty come from balance and efficient use of the body, and follow healthy principles of proper posture and spine alignment, effective postural support, and control of movement in the entire body.

I became a certified Pilates instructor (through the PhysicalMind Institute and the Pilates Method Alliance) and started down my new career path. I found riders of all disciplines interested in improving their riding

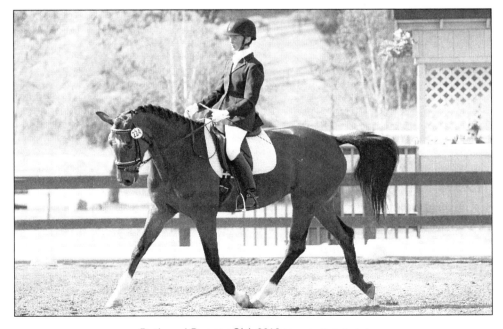

Beth and Donner Girl, 2010 (photo by Cindy Cooke).

skills by improving their fitness, strength, and especially body awareness. Many, like myself, were motivated to learn to ride without pain after injury. After a few years of teaching just Pilates, I started working with clients on their horses—in a program I now call RiderPilates, which includes seminars and clinics linking the skills taught in Pilates to logical use of the body on horseback. Now I am compelled to share my ideas in this book.

Pilates remains an important part of my own personal fitness program, and I believe it has been a huge factor in my ability to continue riding. Since my acute back issues, I've had the great privilege of progressing through the advanced levels of dressage, and, in 2006, I competed successfully at Grand Prix. Now I'm back at the beginning of dressage training with a wonderful young mare. I occasionally experience back flare-ups, but for the most part, by being smart about what I do and using Pilates as described in this book, I rarely need to sit out a day of riding because of my back.

By being smart about what I do and using Pilates as described in this book, I rarely need to sit out a day of riding because of my back.

I continue to learn, train, compete, and enjoy this wonderful sport. I hope you find some tools in this book that will keep you riding for years to come, too.

Overcoming Challenges

Throughout this book in stories titled "My Challenge," you'll read more about my personal riding struggles and how I solved them. In the "Rider's Challenge" stories, you'll discover fictional accounts of my real students' issues and how we worked together to improve their riding effectiveness.

How to Use This Book

This book is designed to give you a systematic, easy-to-understand way to define and address your balance and position issues and equip you with tools to improve your riding effectiveness. I hope to convince you of the importance of posture and body control not only for successful riding, but also for healthy riding. I have created what I think is a logical approach to rider position and function, one based on anatomy and how the human body works. My goal is to clearly present the skills that I think it takes to ride well, and use

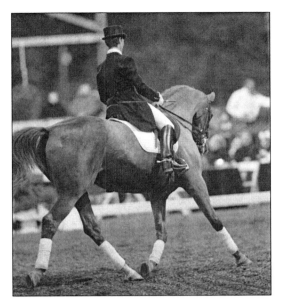

Beth and Bluette, 2006 (Poulsen Photography).

Pilates-based exercises to teach these skills so you can practice and develop these skills off your horse. It is not necessary to read this book cover to cover. You can use it as an overview of rider anatomy and function, or as a reference.

The Rider Checklist

Each chapter focuses on a Rider Checklist element. I developed this checklist to give you an organized and systematic way to assess your balance and position:

- *Keep Mentally Focused*: You consider every step of the ride in terms of you and your horse.
- *Maintain Proper Posture*: You are in correct posture and balance and can maintain this posture and position despite your horse's movement.
- *Control Your Body (Legs and Arms)*: You have control of your legs and arms, and have truly independent aids. Your legs and arms can move with and communicate with your horse without upsetting your balance and position, and your aids can be given in a way that enhance, not interfere with, your horse's way of going.
- *Understand How Your Horse Moves*: You understand the rhythm and basic mechanics of each of your horse's gaits, and translate that into a logical way of moving with your horse at each gait, with appropriately timed aids.

I believe these elements outline the skills you need to be an effective and empathic rider who doesn't get in your horse's way. This checklist was inspired by the Dressage Training Scale (see Table I-1), which sets priorities and goals for horse training. I think it makes sense to have a training scale for us riders, too! When I teach, I use the Rider Checklist to prioritize and organize the issues I see in a rider. You can use this checklist to organize your personal goals separate from your horse's training. And, this checklist is a useful on-the-fly tool to help sort out how you, the rider, could be contributing to difficulties with your horse. For example, if you struggle riding a shoulder-in right, ask, "Am I focused on the movement? Am I in balance? Am I gripping against the movement? Am I in rhythm with my horse, giving appropriately timed aids?" With the Rider Checklist, you can make sure you are doing your part to contribute to the successful execution of a movement or exercise by your horse.

The Rider Checklist elements are all closely related and interdependent. They can, and should, develop coincidently. As your horse's training becomes more advanced, you must develop enhanced precision and control for clear communication. The novice rider starts by mastering all elements of the checklist at the walk, while the advanced rider can refer to the checklist to perfect upper level movements.

Table I-1.

Dressage Training Scale	*Rider Checklist*
Rhythm	Keep Mentally Focused
Relaxation	Maintain Posture and Postural Support
Connection	Control Your Body—Legs
Impulsion	Control Your Body—Arms
Straightness	Understand How Your Horse Moves
Collection	

What Is Pilates?

Pilates is an exercise system named after its originator, Joseph H. Pilates. Pilates developed this system in the early 1900s both to improve his health and to support the health of fellow World War I internees. He developed

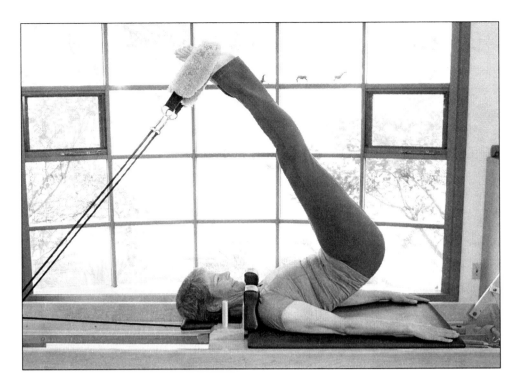

unique equipment that used the variable resistance of springs. In the late 1920s he immigrated to the United States, meeting his wife, Clara, en route, and established the first Pilates studio in New York City.

Joseph Pilates describes the background of his exercise system, which he called "Contrology," in two publications: *Your Health: A Corrective System of Exercising that Revolutionizes the Entire Field of Physical Education* (1934), and *Return to Life Through Contrology* (1945). An array of celebrities came to his studio, and later the dance community embraced his teaching. Later in the twentieth century, the popularity of Pilates spread and studios and training programs opened all over the United States and abroad.

More information about the Pilates system of exercise can be obtained from the Pilates Method Alliance (www.pilatesmethodalliance.org), a not-for-profit organization founded in 1995 to establish certification and continuing education standards for Pilates practitioners.

In Pilates, as in dressage and other riding disciplines, there is more than one take on how to best teach and execute exercises. There is the "New York" or "classical" school that reproduces the work as Joseph Pilates described in his writings and passed down to his students. Another approach (sometimes called "West Coast") takes the Pilates method principles and adapts the

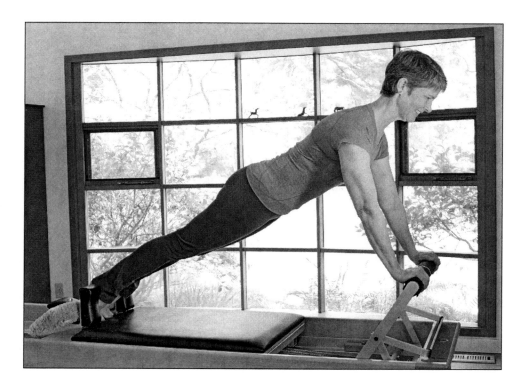

exercises to contemporary science-based notions of movement and spine mechanics. The latter school, endorsed by the Pilates Method Alliance, is the one that I follow.

The important principles of the Pilates exercise program directly translate into tools for the rider to enhance riding ability:

How Pilates Principles Translate into Riders' Tools
- Use mental focus to improve body awareness, movement efficiency, and muscle control:
  A skill required for clear leadership.
- Be aware of neutral spine alignment, or proper posture, throughout the exercises:
  A skill that forms the basis for a balanced position in the saddle.
- Develop the deep abdominal and back muscles to support this posture:
  A skill vital to maintain position, despite your horse's movement.
- Use breath to augment mental focus and centering:
  This technique of using breath is a powerful organizing tool for your body—I call it the rider's half halt!

- Create length, strength, and flexibility in all muscles:
  Promotes suppleness in the shoulder and hip joint muscles while riding, allowing you to move with your horse rather than grip against it.

The principles and exercises I describe in this book are based on the Pilates method. While you do not need Pilates experience to do these exercises, getting input from a Pilates instructor will likely increase the benefit of doing these exercises. Should you seek input from a Pilates instructor, check that your potential instructor has received training in the exercise system and understands any health or movement problems you may have. On the Pilates Method Alliance website you'll find a list of certified instructors. And, at least as of today, you won't find another Pilates program for riders like mine (www.riderpilates.com).

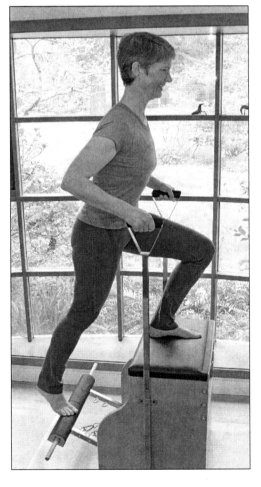

The Pilates exercise system is usually taught in one of two formats: private or semi-private sessions using the unique Pilates equipment, or group mat classes that do not use special equipment but sometimes incorporate simple props.

You may benefit from several one-on-one Pilates sessions with a qualified instructor before participating in a group class. While a private session may be more expensive, the time, money, and effort you devote to learning the exercises correctly is well worth the investment. Sometimes exercises performed incorrectly can be worse for your health than no exercise at all, or at least become a waste of time. Weekly Pilates sessions may be enough, if you commit to practicing between sessions. Twice a week initially will help you learn the program more quickly.

The Pilates principles of movement are taught in some of the simplest exercises of the system. Don't underestimate the benefit of simple movements that support the deep postural trunk muscles, awareness of neutral alignment, and suppleness of the shoulder and hip joint muscles. The most productive Pilates workout requires focus and awareness during each exercise. While the exercises are sometimes difficult to do at first, effective Pilates teaching helps clients develop the skill of complete focus during their workout. This skill can then be applied to any physical activity, including riding.

Given its roots in ballet and dance, some of the movements in the Pilates system are very challenging, even (and in some circumstances, especially) in the mat work. Individuals with significant joint, back, or movement problems, or osteoporosis or osteopenia should avoid these. If you are pushed too fast for your comfort, speak up! The exercises in this system should be challenging (both mentally and physically) but not so difficult that you are struggling. If an exercise causes pain, stop and tell the instructor. You may be doing it incorrectly, or it may be too difficult. Finally, avoid mental and physical fatigue: this is when proper form is lost and the risk of injury is high—just like it is for your horse.

I call the exercises described in this book Pilates based, because while they incorporate Pilates principles and use the Pilates breathing method, some are not part of the original Pilates repertoire. I don't want someone who works with my exercise program to think that if they then take a Pilates mat class, they will have the same experience. There are some overlaps between the programs I have developed and the traditional mat work, but there are also some notable differences. First, I use an exercise ball for many exercises; second, I incorporate balance challenges in the exercises; and third, I adapt some of the exercises to be done asymmetrically, with a single arm or leg, to develop the ability to stay stable in the saddle while giving a single rein or leg aid.

Simple Exercise Equipment

To perform the exercises listed throughout this book, you will need these inexpensive items.

Ball. There are many types and brands of exercise balls available. I have even found some for sale at my local organic grocery store! Purchase a ball that, when fully inflated, enables you to sit with your hip and knee joints level, or with your hip joints slightly higher than your knee joints (Photo

I-1). You should neither feel as if you are sitting precariously high nor feel like you are sitting too low as if in an easy chair. I have found that a 65 cm ball is a good size for many adults.

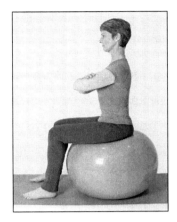

Photo I-1

Mat. Almost any kind of mat will do: the goal is for you to feel comfortable lying on your back or your stomach on the floor. For some, a towel over a carpet is enough.

Weights. I usually start out with 2-pound weights. For some this might be a bit heavy, especially if you have had shoulder injuries or surgery. Most of the exercises that use weights are not really about the weight itself, but about the added challenge to balance conferred by the weight. Start small.

Stretch bands. I use stretchable bands for many of the stretches in this book. These bands come in a variety of weights and degrees of stiffness. I use a band of moderate resistance for the stretches. For all of the leg stretches, however, a large towel that allows you to hold both ends will suffice.

More Nuts and Bolts

Before starting any new exercise program, check with your health care provider. I have done my best to provide written descriptions of the exercises that are clear and safe. However, without feedback from a trained instructor, it can be challenging to do the exercises correctly. If any exercise causes pain, stop—that shouldn't happen. Skip that exercise, or seek feedback from a qualified instructor before proceeding. My mantra for exercising is "mindful, careful, patient, progressive," *not* "no pain, no gain!"

My expertise is in training riders, not horses. Although I have ridden to Grand Prix, I am a *rider* trainer, not a horse trainer. I've had the great pleasure of riding some wonderful horses, but I have worked with many more riders than horses. I place great emphasis on the rider's role in the success of a horse-rider pair. By paying attention to position and balance, the rider is equipped with tools to direct and manage the horse's energy and issues. I certainly recognize the horse has issues of body control, balance, and function! But I will not be addressing these issues per se in this book.

What's more, I give guidance, not medical advice. Although I'm a licensed physician, I do not give medical advice in this book. My goal is to give guidance about the rider's position and function that I think is logical considering how the human body is put together. I learned a great deal about the anatomy and function of the human body from various educational pursuits (medical school, Pilates training, my own injury and rehab programs), but I am not a physiatrist, rehab doctor, orthopedist, or physical therapist. My medical background (and the academic side, for sure) equipped me with analytical tools that help me sort

I place great emphasis on the rider's role in the success of a horse-rider pair. By paying attention to position and balance, the rider is equipped with tools to direct and manage the horse's energy and issues.

out rider issues. It inspired what I hope you find to be straightforward and clear language that describes riding skills in a way that is consistent with human anatomy and movement.

Some of my ideas about how you can best use your body in the saddle are different than those voiced by other authors and riding experts. I believe that this underscores the challenge of using words to describe how to move, especially when there is the complication of another moving animal—your horse! I hope this book offers you some new insight. I apologize if I confuse; I would never be so arrogant as to suggest that my ideas and notions of how things are done on horseback are best. This is my take; I hope there are some useful tools for you.

CHAPTER 1

Keep Mentally Focused

Aproductive training ride requires you to commit positive and unwavering focus to the job at hand. It requires you to organize your thoughts and body movements. Without this commitment, it is difficult to give clear aids to your horse. At best, your vague aids result in a dull horse uninterested and unaffected by your unfocused attempts at communication. At worst, your horse becomes dangerous and spooky, taking over the ride and concerning itself with distractions and events unrelated to you or the ride (Figure 1-1).

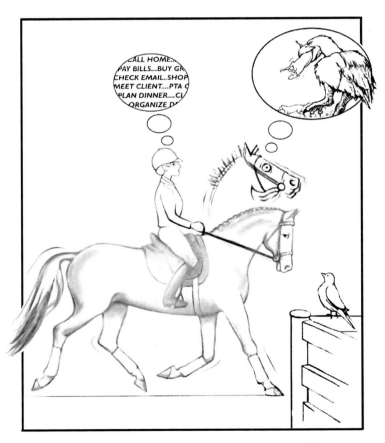

Figure 1-1. Lack of focus on every step of the ride leads to an unfocused and distracted horse.

Finding a clear mind-set is not always easy. Work stresses, family needs, and other responsibilities can conspire to divide your attention during your ride. Your horse perceives this lack of focus as lack of clear leadership. When you settle in the saddle, you owe it to your horse to quiet the chatter in your head and commit all energy to your equine partner. From this place you can fill the role of a clear guide who assesses every step of the ride.

When you settle in the saddle, you owe it to your horse to quiet the chatter in your head and commit all energy to your equine partner.

For this purpose, I developed the 10-minute Preride Warm-Up exercise sequence included in the Suggested Workouts at the end of the book. I designed this short series of simple exercises to get you out of your head and into your body before you sit in the saddle.

The Rider's Challenge: Lack of Focus
Rachel and Mucho

I arrive at Pines Farm as Rachel warms up her 12-year-old Arab gelding, Mucho, in the arena. "I'm concerned about our lesson today," Rachel says, bringing Mucho to a walk. "The hay truck is supposed to arrive soon, and I'm sure he'll be upset and spooked by it."

Rachel looks nervously down the driveway. She cautiously moves Mucho back to the track in a posting trot, occasionally glancing at the road. Mucho, meanwhile, trots hastily with a hollow frame and pricked ears out to the environs. When he looks to the outside of the arena, Rachel snatches at the reins. Mucho gets more hollow and quickens his already-tense trot.

"I hate it when Mucho is so distracted—it is just not fun," Rachel comments.

My challenge today is to help Rachel focus on the job at hand—riding. My goal is to quiet her active imagination and help her keep Mucho *with* her rather than wait for him to spook.

I have Rachel work at the end of the arena, away from potential distractions, and ride some walk-trot transitions. Rachel works on a 20-meter circle, but her transitions are abrupt and disconnected, with Mucho displaying displeasure, tossing his head, and bracing against the bridle.

I am convinced that Rachel's expectation of Mucho getting distracted is guaranteeing that this will happen. I urge her to focus positively on herself, her body, and the rhythm of Mucho's gaits. This helps her think about what is really happening now (not what might happen) and ride Mucho in the way she wants him to go.

I coach Rachel through Pilates breathing exercises while at the walk, guiding her to inhale (breathe in) into the lower ribs, and with each exhale breath to draw her core postural muscles in around her midsection (see Pilates breathing 1 and 2 in this chapter). Each breath releases tension in her arms and shoulder girdle, and her contact with Mucho becomes more elastic. Her body settles into the saddle. I have Rachel count the stepping of Mucho's walking hind legs, which helps her focus on his movement and connect the two of them together. We carry this into walk-trot and trot-walk transitions: Rachel counts the steps in walk, then the quicker steps in trot.

When the hay truck pulls up the driveway, Mucho stops and looks up; Rachel reacts by grabbing the reins with tense shoulders and leaning forward. She quickly recognizes the tension, takes a breath, and gets back to riding. By taking control of her mind and body, she gains better control of Mucho and handles the distraction.

Exercises for Rachel: Pilates breathing 1 and 2, bounce in rhythm 1

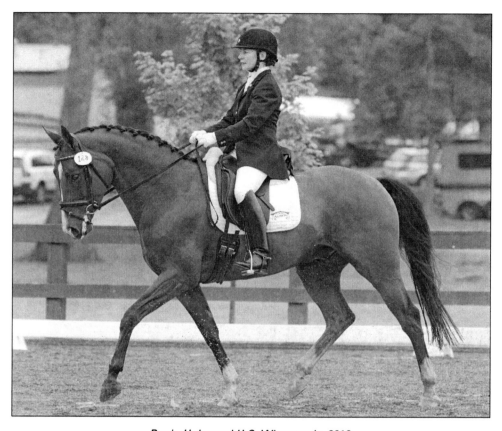

Paula Helm and H.S. Whrapsody, 2010.

Ride Every Step

A simple tool for focusing on every step of your ride is to keep a metronome ticking in your head that matches the rhythm of your horse's gait. At the walk, think of just the stepping of the hind legs so the rhythm is not too fast; at canter, also think of the swing of the hind legs underneath your horse's body as the main beat of the gait (more on this in Chapter 5). Your horse does not have the ability to keep the steadiness of a metronome, but if you focus on keeping the steps-per-minute as regular as possible, three things happen. First, your focus (as in the example with Rachel; see "The Rider's Challenge: Lack of Focus") turns keenly to the present moment-by-moment movement of your horse. Second, you become much more aware that your horse's steps slightly vary but that you can guide your horse to a steadier tempo. Third, by moving closely with it, you become better poised to influence your horse's gait in a positive way.

Past riding experiences, both positive and negative, can profoundly affect your riding mind-set. Fear is a real emotion for many riders, stemming from lack of experience, a past bad experience, or lack of confidence. Work to set reasonable goals for yourself so fear becomes less and less a part of your ride. Seek qualified help for yourself and for your horse so that you learn the skills necessary to get back in control of your rides.

Keen focus will help you solve problems that come up during your ride.

Keen focus will help you solve problems that come up during your ride. Start by becoming aware of what is happening. Why is getting the left lead canter so difficult today? Am I truly committed to going into the canter? Is it my balance? Is it the horse's balance? Do I have suitable impulsion in the trot? Without focus, it is hard to figure out the likely cause of your problem, and you risk repeating it over and over.

Coordinate Your Breathing with Movement

None of us are perfect (oh, really!). On those days when stress makes it difficult to focus on your ride, take some time to settle before you get on your horse. Review Pilates breathing once you are in the saddle. This breathing, your own personal half halt, helps you get out of your busy, noisy head and into your body. It helps settle tension in the shoulders and puts positive energy in your torso to support your balance and posture. If you lose focus during the ride, let this breathing bring you back to your body and your horse's movement. If this fails to shift you into a good riding mind-set, make a note of it. Don't flog yourself: either reduce expectations or go for a trail ride!

Coordinating your breathing with movement is a tool from the Pilates system that promotes mental focus on any physical activity, be it your Pilates workout, work around the house, or riding. It is one of the most valuable tools that I have learned from the Pilates exercise program.

Coordinating your breathing with movement is a tool from the Pilates system that promotes mental focus on any physical activity, be it your Pilates workout, work around the house, or riding. It is one of the most valuable tools that I have learned from the Pilates exercise program. When under time stress, or in the electric and tense environment of a horse show, this breathing helps me slow down and keep my mind and body on the same task. This breathing technique is balancing, organizing, settling; it prepares me for the next exercise, movement, or task. Because of my previous back injury, I use it before I get in my car, lift a bag of groceries, lift my horse's saddle on her back, or lift a bucket of water. The preparatory and organizing feature of this breathing is why I call it the rider's half halt. I use the same technique when riding a half halt on the horse.

Unlike a relaxing method of belly breathing, Pilates breathing is active and energizing. It involves a lateral and outward, not upward, expansion of the rib cage while breathing in (inhaling) and a drawing in of the deep abdominal muscles toward a stable spine while breathing out (exhaling). It is the exhalation phase of the breathing that promotes balance and support, as the technique activates the torso muscles that surround your center of gravity. By using the breath to center, you draw upon the deep muscles of your abdomen and back to improve the balance and stability of your torso as you prepare to move. It draws your focus to your body to optimize effectiveness. The breath keeps you in the moment and enhances riding from the center of your body.

Unlike a relaxing method of belly breathing, Pilates breathing is active and energizing.

Pilates breathing 1
Learn the centering Pilates breathing lying down.

1. Lie on your back on a mat or towel, knees bent, feet flat on the floor about hip joint width apart.

2. Take in a normal breath. As you exhale, let your rib cage drop slightly toward the pelvis, and gently and carefully pull in your abdominal muscles. This movement should feel fluid, not braced (this takes practice). Place your hands on your lower abdomen to feel that the muscles scoop inward. Avoid pressing your abdominal muscles outward, causing a braced feeling in your lower abdomen. This inward movement of the abdominal muscles should not move bones—avoid flattening your back onto the floor.

3. With each inhale breath, work to expand the lower, posterior part of your rib cage, but don't let your upper chest rise up. Keep your abdominals scooped in.

4. With each exhale breath, feel your focus and energy concentrate in the lower abdomen—in your "center."

When done correctly, Pilates breathing should feel like you are creating your own elastic corset of torso support. Your low back should not press into the floor. Your rib cage should not push off the floor. Your spine and pelvis bones should not move. The engagement of your deep abdominal and back muscles should create a feeling of the rib cage and pelvis being elastically connected and knitted together. But again, when done correctly, no bones move. The breath just firms up the muscles around your midsection.

If you are having trouble keeping your abdominals scooped in as you breathe in, place your hands on the sides of your ribs. As you inhale, imagine your ribs swinging outward, or laterally, toward your hands. In fact, this is the way ribs are intended to move: like a bucket handle swinging out to the side as you breathe in.

This method of breathing is different from a relaxing "breathing into the belly" type of breath. Belly breathing, in which the abdominal muscles are released as you breathe in, offers less support during the inhale breath, making it less suitable for activity. With Pilates breathing, the goal is to use the exhale breath to activate and connect to the deep muscles of your lower abdomen and back so they are "on" and ready to support you during movement. Breathing into the lateral and posterior rib cage allows continued abdominal and back support during inhalation. As a result, you maintain unwavering postural support and balance throughout breathing.

Practicing Pilates breathing while you are lying on the floor helps you feel whether or not the bones of your spine move while you breathe. It is not the goal for your spine alignment to change.

Pilates breathing 2
Learn the centering Pilates breathing while sitting.

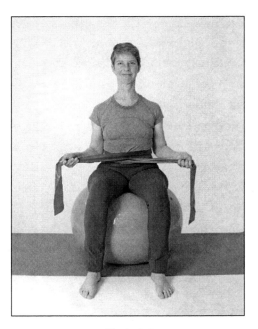

Photo 1-1

1. Sit upright in a chair or on an exercise ball, feet flat on the floor, hip joint width apart. Align your body so that your shoulders are over your pelvis (more about alignment in Chapter 2).

2. Wrap a towel or stretchy band around your midsection, cross it in front of your body, and hold one end in each hand (Photo 1-1). If you lack a stretchy band, you can use your hands: place one hand on your abdomen and one hand on your back.

3. Take an easy breath in. As you exhale, gently pull on the ends of the band or towel so it squeezes around your middle. Or, imagine your hand on your abdomen pressing toward your hand on your back. As in Pilates breathing 1, pull your abdominal muscles inward as you breathe out, and allow your ribs to drop down and in slightly (but don't round your body forward). It should feel as if you are making the space inside the towel or stretchy band smaller.

4. As you breathe in again, keep muscle tone in your lower torso, expanding your ribs out to the side.

Practice this breathing technique many times a day, and it will gradually become more natural. Learning the breathing as you sit upright makes the exercise more relevant to riding. Breathe when you are stressed and harried, and before you need to lift something. Practice in your car and use it to divert your mind from annoying traffic: breathe and center and take satisfaction that you are learning to organize your body and keep your brain quiet and focused—even in frustrating driving situations. Begin each ride by taking a few breaths in the saddle to help you feel connected to the middle of your body. Soon it will become a positive habit of preparing and balancing your body.

My Challenge: Fear of Pain

I am not the bravest rider—not at all. Much of my concern stems from not wanting to hurt myself. I am sympathetic to how unnerving the unreliable movements of a horse can be. You won't find me riding the hottest horse in the barn! So I feel I can speak confidently about how fitness and body control can help you deal with riding fears.

As Pilates improved my fitness and balance, I found that if my horse spooked, I was much better able to stay with him without even really having to think about it. A few positive experiences like this helped reduce my anxiety about the possibility of spooks (and back injury).

I cannot underscore enough the power of Pilates breathing and using core muscles to anchor yourself in the saddle. On windy days, for example, I expect that my horse might move unpredictably, so I prepare in three ways: First, I assess whether I will likely have a productive ride, given the circumstances. Second, I choose a part of the arena where spooking is less likely, especially in the warm-up phase of my ride. And third, I commit a great deal of focus to keeping my body centered, balanced, and in the saddle by breathing and counting my horse's steps.

Bounce in rhythm 1

*This exercise brings precision to your perception of tempo
and is a great warm-up exercise.*

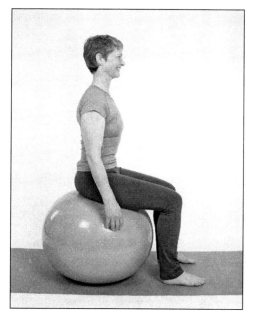

Photo 1-2

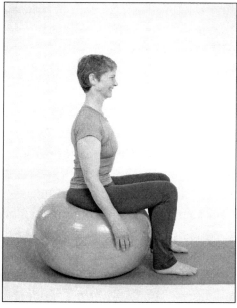

Photo 1-3

1. Set a metronome to about 92 to 98 beats per minute, or put on some music with a similar beat.

2. Sit on an exercise ball in upright posture. Bounce on the ball to the beat of the metronome or music (Photos 1-2 and 1-3).

3. Work to control your tempo so that you stay precisely with the beat. You'll find it is not as easy as it sounds: it is challenging to keep absolutely steady with the beat. This practice on the ball will help you guide your horse to a steady tempo.

4. Work to land the same way on the ball each time; this is also harder than it sounds, but it will help you develop skills to keep a steady position on your moving horse.

My Challenge: Learning to Focus Inward

Pilates taught me how to turn my focus inward to feel what happens when I move. Before, if I lifted weights or did a leg exercise, it would just be about the arms lifting weights or the legs pressing a bar. With practice, I could feel the coordination that happened in my body to accomplish an arm or leg movement. With this awareness, movements became more balanced and fluid and less jerky and disruptive. And, movement done with this awareness was less likely to bother my back.

This focus translates to my riding. With awareness I can note how my body moves on the horse, at times in undesirable ways. Awareness has improved my balance and timing so I can stay with my horse and give subtle aids rather than aids that are jerky and disruptive, both to me and to my horse.

With your mind now engaged on movement, next we'll pursue specifics of posture and spine alignment, the basis of a correct and functional riding position.

CHAPTER 2

Maintain Proper Posture

The basis for a balanced and stable position and effective riding is good posture and muscular support of this posture. Correct posture provides the foundation for efficient riding and organized management of the horse's energy. While proper posture creates an elegant position, it is not just about looking good! Proper posture is a healthy position for the spine and the position from which we can most easily balance and move with efficiency.

Riding with correct and stable posture allows arm and leg muscle suppleness, and facilitates clear communication with the horse. The Pilates exercise system teaches good posture and supple arm and leg movement. It uses the stability of good posture and torso control as a steppingstone for more and more challenging exercises—just like dressage.

What Is Balance?

Balance describes a state of equilibrium, or stability and steadiness, that is maintained despite movement input. Our life experiences teach us to deal with unbalancing situations such as walking on rough ground, carrying an infant with one arm, or putting on a shoe. While riding, however, you are expected to sit "quietly" on a constantly moving surface—the horse! Moreover, that "surface" does not always move predictably. It is no wonder that many find maintaining balance on their horse and coordinating aids is terribly challenging. The moving horse presents a huge threat to balance. A sudden spook can overwhelm balance in the best of riders and lead to a fall, but failures in balance can occur even during planned movements and transitions. A balanced rider seeks her own self-carriage, with her torso steadily positioned over the horse's movement. The balance must be so secure that the rider feels like a legless doll in the saddle. From this place, suppleness in the hip and shoulder joint muscles is possible, and the ideal image of horse and rider moving as one can emerge.

Riding in balance confers a sense of being centered, physically and mentally.

Physically being centered means riding with the middle of your body as your base of support. It means riding with correct posture and postural support, and with movement controlled from the area around your center of gravity. It promotes riding with awareness and balance.

A concrete way to define your balanced center is to equate it to the physical location of your center of gravity. The center of gravity is a theoretical place in the body where body weight is concentrated or evenly distributed. In the upright human, this point is in the middle of the torso, roughly just above the pelvis, a little below the belly button, and just in front of the junction of the lumbar spine and sacrum. For our discussions, the precise location of the center of gravity is academic. What is much more important is recognizing the power of riding from this general place within your body. This place should be the starting point for your aids, assisted by your arms and legs.

Your balanced center can be viewed as your "movement processing center." Energy from your moving horse is put into your body. (If you don't believe me, imagine your horse galloping to a jump and then stopping: if you are not balanced and prepared to deal with this sudden change in energy, your body continues over the jump—alone!) A centered rider is not put off balance by this energy, does not interfere with the horse's movement, and can manipulate this energy to direct and improve the horse's way of going. A stable position of your torso with support around your center of gravity facilitates your core (or center) being your energy processing center, or movement processing center.

Directing your horse by considering how the core of your body interfaces with its energy (more forward, more up, more sideways) helps you balance and communicate with your horse in a way that you feel you are moving with your horse, not just sitting on top of it. You are balanced and in self-carriage, owning every step of the ride. This idea is fundamental to how I apply Pilates to riding and inspired the energy management diagram (Figure 2-1).

For many, accessing and riding from the movement processing center is not a natural or instinctive way to think of riding: it needs to be learned. This is not surprising, however, as our hand-eye-dominated life tends to draw us away from our body's movement processing center, allowing the sometimes overbearing thought processing center (brain and upper body) to dominate. This leads to a stiff position, with shoulders and arms taking over the ride. When we keep movement control in our center, we enjoy improved balance, coordination, and grace. Consider a ballerina: her centered movement

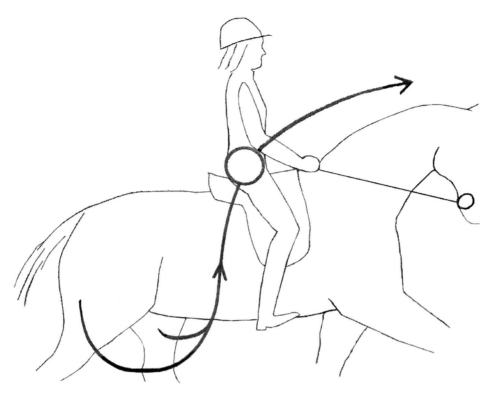

Figure 2-1. Energy comes from the horse and passes through the rider's center, where it is directed as desired by the rider: forward, upward, or sideways.

allows extreme precision of balance so she can remain tall and steady on the toes of one foot while creating graceful arcing movements with her arms. This is only possible with a foundation of balance from her center or core.

Correct and stable posture has the additional benefit of conferring a powerful sense of self, the mental aspect of being balanced and centered. From here, you become a proactive rider, creating the ride you want rather than reacting to what your horse does. Your physical center can be a place of peace in your body. Pilates breathing, as discussed in Chapter 1, draws your focus to this center. Breathing in this way helps quiet a busy head (thought processing center working overtime) and reminds you of your movement, or energy, processing center.

Finding good posture and being centered and balanced on horseback starts with an understanding of basic anatomy—just enough to help you find your correct spine alignment and support it with the muscular tools within your body.

The Rider's Challenge: Organize Riding from the Center
Stephanie and Atticus

Stephanie, a new rider at my clinic, rides over on her spicy, 16-years-young Thoroughbred gelding, Atticus. I ask her about her lesson goals.

"I don't know," Stephanie replies. "I'm sure I need to work on a lot of things."

Stephanie moves onto the rail with high-headed Atticus and picks up a posting trot. Atticus is irregular in his tempo, causing Stephanie to alternately fall back as he moves off into his quick trot and fall forward when he slows down in response to her pulling on the reins. This pattern repeats with Stephanie alternately kicking to keep him in trot, falling back as he trots forward, then pulling on the reins to slow him down and falling forward as he does. He remains tense and snorting at the environment, while Stephanie struggles for constancy.

Stephanie needs to gain mastery over her own focus and balance to control Atticus's trot. She must buy into riding every step and riding for the trot she wants. That is, become a proactive, rather than a reactive, rider. She must develop a clear sense of balance around her center, and ride from her center rather than just from her arms and legs.

I teach Stephanie the Pilates breathing technique so she can get a sense of her source of balance coming from the middle of her body. With one hand, I gently press against her lower abdomen, bringing her abdominal wall closer to her spine, without rounding her back. My other hand presses against her low back to keep it in a stable position. I urge her to keep her abdominal muscles engaged and pulling inward to help stabilize her balance, and to imagine there is a "hum" of energy coming from these muscles supporting her body during the ride.

Back on the rail, Stephanie practices her breathing to engage her core muscles. She rides some walk-halt transitions, focusing on using her breath to stabilize her body during the halt and to prepare her body to move forward with Atticus into the walk. In the trot,

I encourage her to keep her core muscles "humming" and to feel her center move forward and back in the posting trot. She counts a steady tempo to stabilize her horse's tempo. Atticus continues his speeding up and slowing down cycles, but Stephanie's body position stays fairly steady and her aids become less dramatic and destabilizing.

Exercises for Stephanie: Pilates breathing 1 and 2; bounce in rhythm 1; pelvic rocking on ball, front to back; pelvic rocking on ball, side to side; bounce in rhythm 3—toe tapping

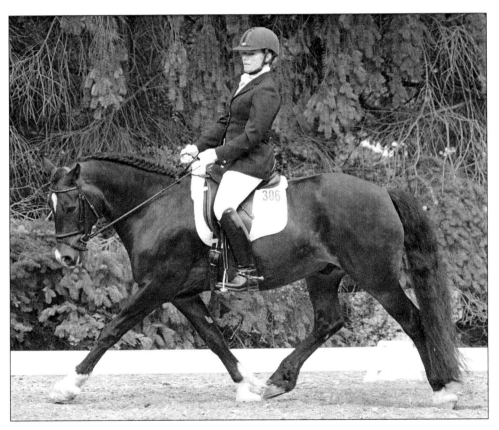

Lisa Boyer and Winterlake Gulliver (owned by Yvonne Billera), 2010.

Anatomy of Posture: Bones

Posture refers to the alignment of the spine, and good posture is correct spine alignment. The spine is a series of stacked bones, or vertebrae. It extends from the base of the skull to the sacrum, and, among other functions, provides the rigid support of our upright body position. Figure 2-2 shows that these vertebrae of the spine are not stacked in a straight line, but form curves. Seven vertebrae form a curve at the neck or cervical spine; twelve form a curve at the mid back or thoracic spine, where the ribs are attached; and five form a curve at the low back, or lumbar spine. The last five vertebrae of the spine are fused to form the sacrum, the back part of the pelvis. While the precise degree of spine curvature varies from person to person, allowing and supporting these curves preserves proper spine function and health. This alignment is called "neutral spine alignment" and defines correct posture. It is the basis of a correct position in the saddle. Understanding this position of your spine is a huge part of Pilates-based exercise.

Neutral spine is the most efficient alignment of your spine for balance. Stated another way, if you are not in neutral spine alignment, your body must compensate somehow for your less-than-ideal posture, which can result in unnecessary tension in your shoulders, back, or legs. Finding and keeping good posture improves your body function and movement.

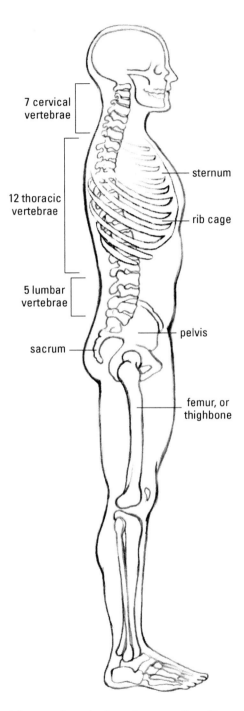

7 cervical
vertebrae

sternum

12 thoracic
vertebrae

rib cage

5 lumbar
vertebrae

pelvis

sacrum

femur, or
thighbone

*Figure 2-2. Alignment of the vertebrae in the spine, standing. Note the curves in the seven
vertebrae that comprise the neck or cervical spine, the twelve vertebrae of the thoracic
spine (ribs attached), and the five vertebrae of the lumbar spine. The spine ends at the
sacrum. Proper posture allows for these curves in the spine.*

The Vertebrae

Each vertebra of the spine has a cushioning disk between it and its neighbors above and below. These disks, as well as other bony joint connections between vertebrae, allow movement so we can rotate our spine, as well as bend it forward, backward, and sideways. However, these joints become stressed and worn out with repeated and excess movements, or prolonged periods of time in postures other than neutral alignment. Back pain or nerve impingement can result. So good posture not only is beautiful and elegant (Figure 2-3), but it also helps preserve the health of your spine.

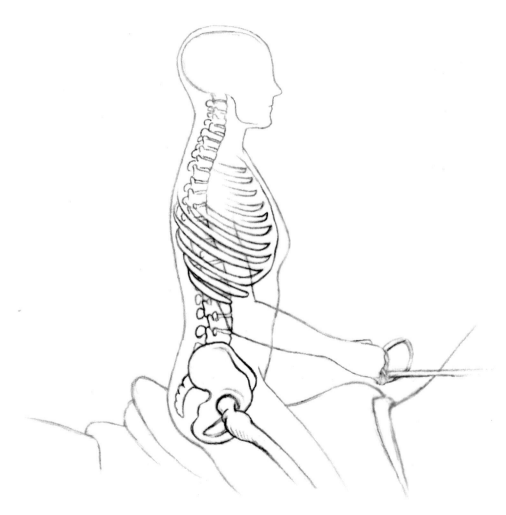

*Figure 2-3. Proper spine alignment, or posture, in the saddle.
Note that the curves in the neck, thoracic area, and lumbar spine
are preserved, and the rib cage is aligned over the pelvis.*

The Pelvis and Rib Cage

The spine ends in five fused vertebrae that form the sacrum or the back of the pelvis. The pelvis (Figure 2-4), for our purposes, will be considered a ring of bone that connects the trunk of the body to the legs. The pelvis provides support for our abdominal and pelvic organs, and via the hip joints disperses the downward force of our body weight onto the legs, and absorbs concussion from the contact of our legs to the ground. The seat bones, or "ischial tuberosities," form the base or lowest part of the pelvis. These are the bony prominences upon which we sit and are most obvious when seated on a hard chair. When in neutral spine in the saddle, the ischial tuberosities point roughly downward. The bony prominences of the right and left sides of the pelvis in the front of the body are called the "anterior superior iliac spines" or ASIS. This part is sometimes called the "hip." I will refer to this part of the pelvis in some of the exercises.

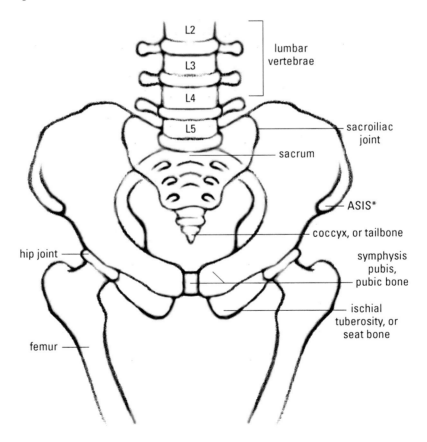

*Figure 2-4. The pelvis is essentially a ring of bone that connects the single column of stacked vertebrae to the legs. *anterior superior iliac spine*

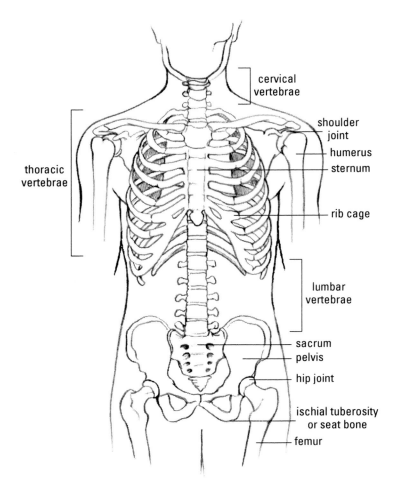

Figure 2-5. The ribs attach to the thoracic vertebrae; the spine
ends in the sacrum, which forms the back of the pelvis. The pelvis
disperses the weight of the body onto the legs at the hip joints, and
also disperses the concussion of walking.

We sit on the pelvis in the saddle. In fact, distribution of our weight
over the floor of the pelvis can be used to reference our posture and body
position. The pelvic floor consists of the muscles and tissues that form the
bottom of the pelvis. It is through these tissues that the urethra, vagina, and
anus pass. The pelvic floor is shaped somewhat like a diamond, with the arch
of the pubic bone in front, the tailbone/sacrum toward the back, and a seat
bone on either side. The precise location of body weight over the pelvic floor
will depend upon your unique anatomy, the shape of the twist of your saddle,
and your horse's anatomy. After being guided to neutral spine alignment in

the saddle, note the distribution of weight over your pelvic floor. Alterations in this weight distribution during your ride can inform you of changes in your body position, alignment, and balance.

The rib cage (Figure 2-5) provides bony protection for our vital organs, the heart and lungs. The ribs connect to the thoracic vertebrae in the spine.

The relationship between the pelvis and rib cage in the front of the body can provide important landmarks for spine alignment. Any change in spine alignment will, by definition, alter the distance between the rib cage and the pelvis (Figure 2-6 A-C). This is most easily detected in the front of the body by considering the distance between the bottom ribs and the ASIS. If a rider maintains neutral spine alignment while moving or riding, this distance will stay fairly stable. If spine alignment changes, this distance also changes.

It takes some time and practice to understand where neutral spine alignment is in your body and what it feels like while riding. First, understand what it feels like off your horse, and then, with mirrors or feedback from someone on the ground, learn what it feels like on your horse. Neutral spine alignment on horseback puts your body in the correct shoulder-hip-heel alignment referred to in many discussions of rider position, and is the anatomic basis for this ideal position (Figure 2-3).

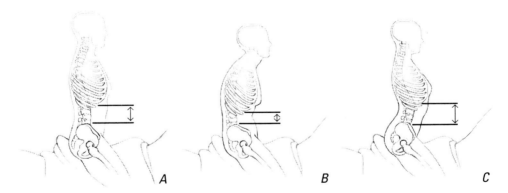

Figure 2-6. A. Neutral alignment has a defined distance between ribs and pelvis.
B. A rounded, or flexed, posture results in a decreased distance between ribs
and pelvis in front of the body compared to neutral spine alignment.
C. An arched, or extended, posture results in an increased distance between ribs
and pelvis in front of the body compared to neutral spine alignment.

Find neutral spine
By lying on the floor, you can feel the alignment of the vertebrae and perceive the normal curves in your spine.

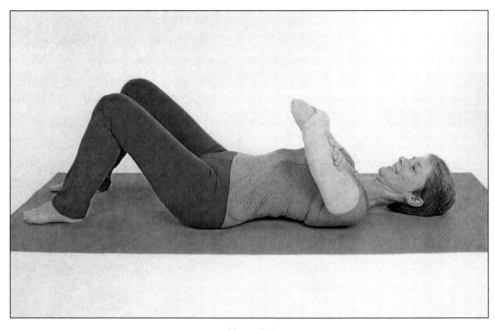

Photo 2-1

1. Lie on the floor or a mat, knees bent, feet flat on the floor hip joint width apart (Photo 2-1).

2. Release the muscles of your back and let the weight of your body sink onto the floor (without pressing or forcing any part of your back onto the floor).

3. Note where you feel the weight of your body touch the floor. When the spine is in neutral alignment with its normal curves, your weight contacts the floor in three places: at the back of your pelvis or sacrum, around your shoulder and shoulder blades, and at the back of your head. There is usually little weight contacting the floor behind your waist and behind your neck.

This describes the normal curves of your spine. Everyone is slightly different, but the point is that your back is not completely flat.

Pelvic rocking supine

Explore changing your spine alignment
with small movements of your pelvis.

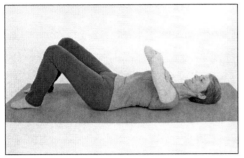
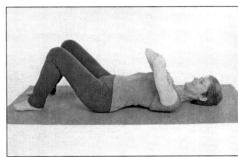

Photo 2-2   Photo 2-3

1. Lie on the floor or a mat, knees bent, feet flat on the floor hip joint width apart, in neutral alignment (Photo 2-1).

2. Take an easy inhale breath, breathing into your lateral rib cage.

3. On the exhale breath, scoop in your abdominal muscles to rock the top of your pelvis *toward* the floor (posterior pelvic tilt, or pelvic tuck), flattening your low back (Photo 2-2).

4. On the next inhale breath, rock the top of your pelvis *away* from the floor (anterior pelvic tilt), arching your back slightly so that your low back comes off the floor (Photo 2-3).

5. Slowly alternate flattening and arching your low back 6 to 8 times, inhaling as you arch your spine, exhaling as you flatten your spine onto the floor.

6. Gradually decrease your range of motion until, like a pendulum, your low back comes to rest. This position is likely very close to your neutral spine alignment.

7. When your spine is in neutral alignment, the plane defined by the three points of your pubic bone and right and left ASIS (the prominent bones of the front of your pelvis) will be parallel to the floor (Photo 2-1). When you stand, or sit in the saddle, this plane will be perpendicular to the floor.

Once you have found neutral spine alignment, or good posture, you need to keep your spine in this position despite being on a moving horse! Support of good posture on horseback not only keeps your spine in a healthy position, but also provides the most efficient position from which to achieve balance.

Anatomy of Posture: Muscles

Balance and postural support come from the deepest muscle layers of the torso. These muscles are designed to support our upright posture throughout our daily activities and do so quite efficiently. These muscles, called the slow-twitch muscles, have a metabolism that supports a low level of constant activity for prolonged periods. Their metabolic machinery works at a steady rate, using oxygen efficiently to fuel their daylong work. This makes them different from the fast-twitch muscles, designed to work at high levels of activity for short periods of time. Balance, an integral part of our daily lives (but often taken for granted), relies upon a constant low level of support from our slow-twitch postural muscles. Running for the bus, on the other hand, relies on the fast-twitch, sprinting muscles of our legs. Consider the fatigue you experience from sprinting: fast-twitch muscles get this job done, but at a price! While riding, for balance we need to access the efficient postural muscles, not the fatigue-inducing leg muscles.

The postural muscles of the torso include the deep abdominal muscles and the deep back muscles.

Abdominal Muscles

There are four layers of muscles in the abdominal wall. From deep within the body to the more superficial, they include the transversus abdominis, the internal oblique, the external oblique, and the rectus abdominis.

The two deepest layers of abdominal muscles are the most important for postural support.

The transversus abdominis (Figure 2-7) muscle fibers run transversely, or across the body. Since muscle fibers only shorten when they contract, using this abdominal muscle results in a pulled-in abdominal wall or belly, making your midsection flat. It pulls your middle to a smaller diameter (like when you are trying to fit into jeans a size too small). Because this muscle essentially wraps all around the midsection, activating this muscle creates a corset-like support of your spine and torso. It is the primary muscle activated in the Pilates breathing 1 and 2 exercises described in Chapter 1. Pulling in

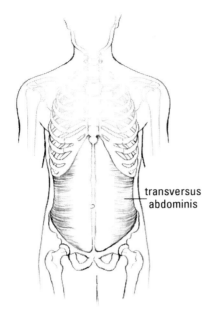

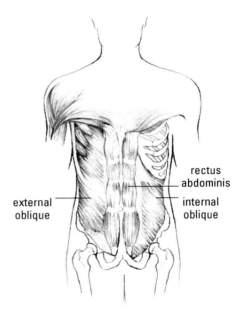

Figure 2-7. The transversus abdominis
muscle is the deepest abdominal wall
muscle. Its action pulls the abdominal wall
flat and is important for postural support.

Figure 2-8. The internal oblique, external
oblique, and rectus abdominis muscles.
The obliques rotate, side bend, and
forward bend (flex) the trunk.

the abdominal muscles on the exhale breath activates this transversus abdominis muscle and stabilizes the spine, posture, and balance, preparing you
for the next moment of your ride.

The internal oblique is the second deepest muscle layer and is one of
three muscles shown in Figure 2-8. Its fibers run from the rim of the pelvis
to the rib cage. When just the right or left internal oblique muscle contracts,
it causes side bending or rotation to that side. The muscle can also resist
these same movements to the other side. When both right and left internal
oblique muscles contract, they, along with the external oblique muscles, pull
the rib cage closer to the pelvis, causing flexion or forward bending of the
spine. As well, these muscles resist spine extension or arch.

The most superficial abdominal muscle, the rectus abdominis, is less
important for postural support and balance. This muscle, when developed,
creates the "washboard abs" appearance. While some may desire this look,
development of this muscle does little for posture, body support, or balance.

Back Muscles

The deep muscles of the back are as important for postural support and balance as the deep abdominal muscles. There are many layers of back muscle (Figure 2-9). The deepest layers, the multifidi, span only one or two vertebrae. Back muscle activation pulls the spine into an arch, or extension. Also, the back muscles resist forward bending.

Your Muscles Create a Corset of Support for Posture

From these muscle descriptions you can imagine how balanced use of the transversus abdominis, internal obliques, and the deep back muscles work together to move your spine in all directions as well as to stabilize your spine in good posture despite movement forces from all directions. Like a corset around your middle, these muscles create a toned elastic support system to preserve alignment of your spine. This muscular support provides the tool for body stability and balance. Your spine stays stable despite the input of movement forces from your horse.

Essentially all Pilates exercises teach you to access and improve function of the deep muscles of the abdomen and back and thus develop these strong and efficient tools for balance. Some exercises directly strengthen these muscles through movement, while others challenge the ability of these muscles to maintain alignment and spine stability during leg and/or arm movements. Both approaches are valuable. You develop sufficient muscle connection, strength, and coordination to stay in good posture and balance on your moving horse, and use of an arm or leg aid does not disrupt this balance. Truly independent aids are then possible.

Some recommend pressing the abdominal muscles out to achieve a stable body position. I do not believe this is the best strategy for supporting stability in the context of movement, which is what we have on horseback, and for that matter, during much of our day-to-day activities. Along with many physiotherapists and spine experts, I advise using these muscles as they are designed—to come inward toward the center of the body, offering a strong elastic support for movement in good alignment (see "Abdominal Muscles: Pull In or Push Out?" in this chapter).

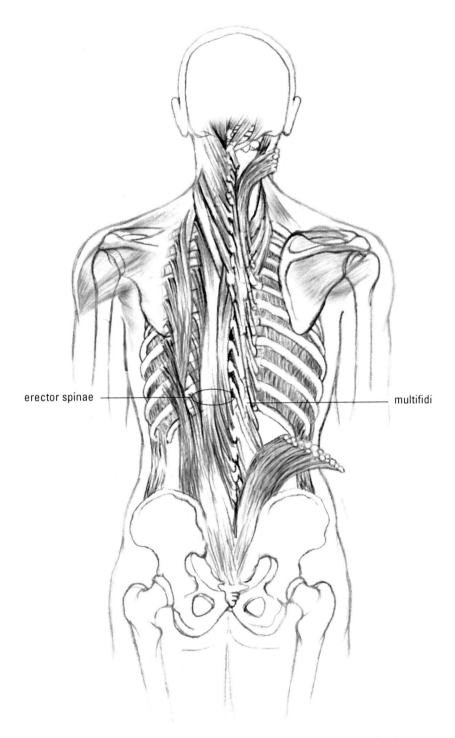

erector spinae — multifidi

Figure 2-9. The back muscles cause spine extension, or move the spine into an arch.
The deepest layers (multifidi) are most important for spine stability.

Pelvic rocking on ball, front to back
*Control the position of your pelvis with
your abdominal and back muscles.*

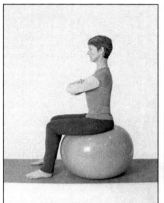 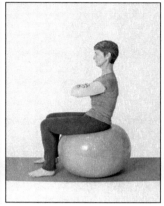 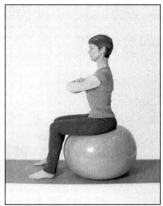

Photo 2-4   *Photo 2-5*   *Photo 2-6*

1. Sit upright, in neutral spine alignment, on an exercise ball with your feet flat on the floor, hip joint width apart (Photo 2-4). You may need a colleague or a mirror to check that you are in neutral spine alignment, with your shoulders aligned over your pelvis and your seat bones pointing downward.

2. Take an easy inhale breath and as you exhale, scoop in your abdominal muscles to rock your pelvis into a tuck, pointing your seat bones toward your heels and rounding your low back (Photo 2-5). Allow your shoulders to follow the movement; do not lean back.

3. Inhale and use your deep back muscles to rock your pelvis back so that there is a slight arch in your spine, and your seat bones point toward the back of the ball (Photo 2-6).

4. Exhale and tuck your pelvis under again, and inhale to point your seat bones behind you.

5. Rock back and forth between these positions 6 to 8 times, gradually settling to the middle of the movement, in neutral spine alignment.

Concentrate on using your torso muscles to move your pelvis front and back. Try not to use your leg muscles to move your pelvis. This exercise should help you feel grounded with your weight centered over your pelvis, efficiently balanced on the exercise ball.

Abdominal curls
Strengthen your deep abdominal muscles with this simple exercise.

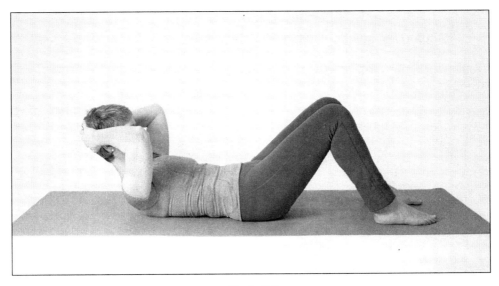

Photo 2-7

1. Lie on the floor in neutral spine alignment, knees bent, feet flat on the floor hip joint width apart.

2. Place your hands behind your head or neck.

3. Take a normal breath in and as you exhale, scoop in your lower abdomen and peel your upper body off the floor in a curl. Inhale as you roll back down (Photo 2-7).

4. Repeat 8 to 10 times.

Keep your abdominal muscles scooped in as you curl up. Keep your fingers soft behind your head; don't pull yourself up with your arms. Avoid pushing your low back into the mat by tucking your pelvis. Allow your back to lengthen. Feel your neck lengthen as you round your head forward in the curl, leading with your forehead. Curl up until just the bottom of your shoulder blades touches the floor, or less. Keep the movement smooth, not jerky. Keep breathing throughout the movement. Feel how your rib cage comes closer to your pelvis during the exercise.

Done this way, this exercise strengthens the deep abdominal muscles. If your abdominal muscles bulge out, you are using the more superficial abdominal wall muscles, making the exercise less useful.

Abdominal curls variation 1
Changing leg position adds difficulty to the abdominal curl exercise.

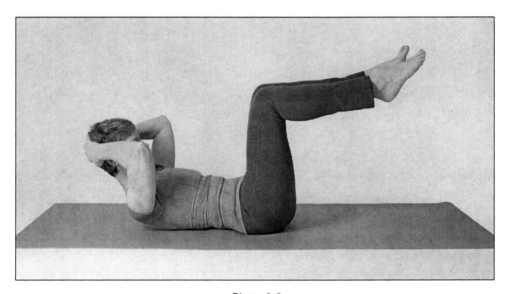

Photo 2-8

To make the abdominal curl exercise more challenging, position your legs in a tabletop position with your hip and knee joints at right angles (Photo 2-8). Perform the exercise as described above.

Abdominal curls sustained

*To add more challenge to the abdominal curl exercise,
perform a single sustained curl.*

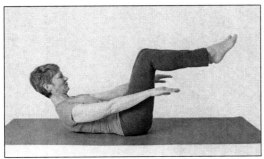
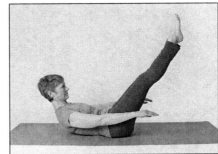

Photo 2-9   Photo 2-10

1. Lie on the floor in neutral spine alignment, knees bent, feet flat on the floor hip joint width apart.

2. Place your arms by your side.

3. Take a normal breath in and as you exhale, scoop in your lower abdomen and peel your upper body off the floor in a curl, reaching your arms forward toward your shins. Place your legs in tabletop position *or* straighten your legs onto a high diagonal line (Photos 2-9 and 2-10).

4. Keep the curled position as you breathe in and out. Try to breathe into your posterior rib cage so your inhale breath does not cause you to lose any of the curl. Each time you exhale, pull your abdominal muscles inward.

5. Repeat for 8 to 10 breaths.

If your neck gets sore during the sustained curl, try to curl up a bit more or support your head with your hands. Keep an inward pull on your abdominal muscles, and avoid letting the abdominal muscles bulge outward. Extend your legs straight onto a high diagonal line only if your abdominal muscles are strong enough to support your low back.

Crisscross
*This abdominal curl variation puts greater demand
on the oblique abdominal muscles.*

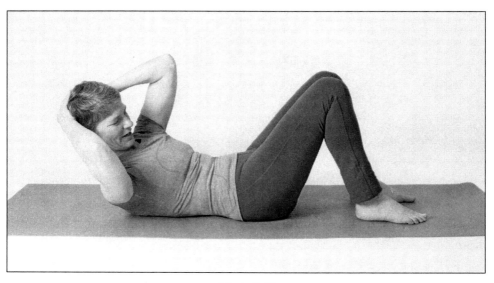

Photo 2-11

1. Lie on the floor in neutral spine alignment, knees bent, feet flat on the floor hip joint width apart.

2. Place your hands behind your head or neck.

3. Take a normal breath in and as you exhale, scoop in your lower abdomen and peel your upper body off the floor in a curl. At the top of the curl, add a rotation of your torso to the right, as if you were bringing your left rib cage toward your right pelvis (Photo 2-11). Inhale as you roll back down.

4. Repeat the curl rotating toward the left, bringing your right rib cage toward your left pelvis.

5. Repeat 6 to 8 times each direction.

Coordinate your breath with the movement. Avoid lifting your head with your arms, but feel your abdominal muscles pull your rib cage toward your pelvis and then add the rotation from your abdominals, not your arms. The focus is on curling up and then rotating.

Crisscross sustained

Add more challenge to the crisscross exercise by sustaining the curl.

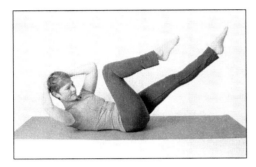
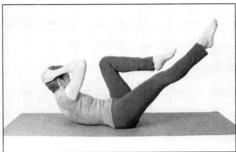

Photo 2-12   *Photo 2-13*

1. Lie on the floor in neutral spine alignment, knees bent, feet flat on the floor hip joint width apart.

2. Place your hands behind your head or neck.

3. Take a normal breath in and as you exhale, scoop in your lower abdomen and peel your upper body off the floor in a curl. Position your left leg straight at a 45-degree angle, or high diagonal, and place your right leg in tabletop position. Rotate your torso toward your right knee (Photo 2-12).

4. Reverse the leg positions and the rotation in your torso (Photo 2-13).

5. Breathe out each time you rotate and breathe in as you switch your leg position.

6. Repeat 8 times in each direction.

As with the other abdominal curl exercises, avoid lifting your head and rotating your body with your arms; use your abdominal muscles to draw the rib cage to the pelvis and then to one side. Focus more on the *up* part of the curl, not the turning part of the curl. Carefully place your legs in their correct positions, feeling your straight leg reach out of the hip joint. Keep your leg position under control.

Spine extension on mat
This exercise strengthens the muscles of your mid- and upper back.

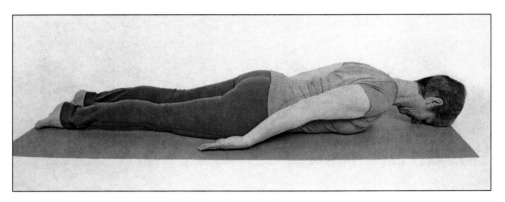

Photo 2-14

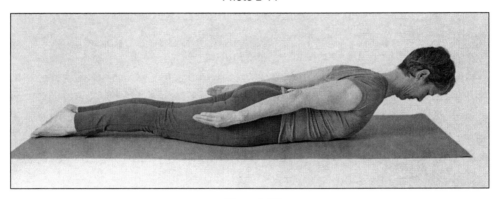

Photo 2-15

1. Lie on the floor on your stomach, resting your forehead on a towel if needed for comfort.

2. Place your arms by your sides with palms up (Photo 2-14).

3. Take an easy inhale breath, and on the exhale breath, pull your abdominal wall up off the floor (this should not be a visible movement—just a pulling in of your abdomen to support your lumbar spine).

4. On the next inhale breath, bring your shoulder blades together and slowly lift your upper body off the floor. The muscles to lift your upper body should be the deep mid- and upper back muscles (Photo 2-15).

5. Exhale as you rest your upper body back down.

6. Repeat 4 to 6 times.

Initiate the movement with your shoulder blades coming down your back toward the center of your body, not from your neck (Photo 2-16). Feel that you keep your head and neck in alignment with the rest of your spine. Feel as if your back is getting longer, reaching away from your pelvis. If this exercise causes low back pain, reduce the range of motion and seek support from your scooped-in deep abdominal muscles, or avoid the exercise until you can get expert feedback.

Follow the exercise set with a back stretch.

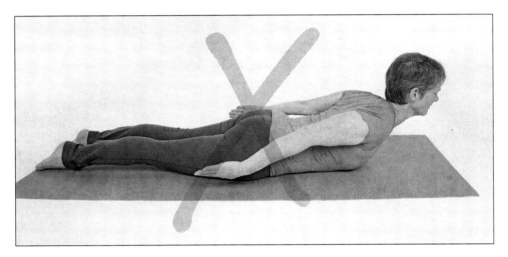

Photo 2-16

Back stretch

This stretch provides relief for the back muscles after they have worked.

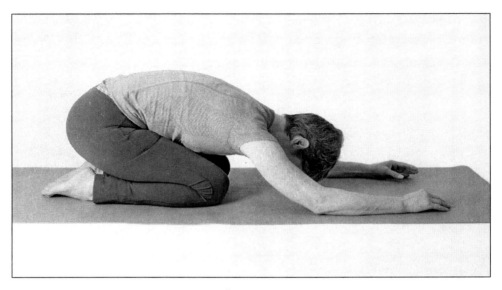

Photo 2-17

1. Start on your hands and knees. Sit back toward your heels and lower your forehead toward the mat (Photo 2-17).

2. Either reach your arms overhead, resting your hands on the floor, or keep them by your sides.

3. Use your breath to stretch your back muscles. As you breathe in, feel how expanding your rib cage stretches your back muscles. As you exhale, focus on scooping in the abdominal muscles to support the stretch of your low back muscles. Hold for several breaths.

4. Walk your hands over to your right side, stretching the left side of your body. Breathe into the left rib cage 2 to 3 times to facilitate the stretch.

5. Walk your hands over to your left side, stretching the right side of your rib cage.

Spine stretch forward

This exercise provides a stretch to your back and improves awareness of the location of your rib cage in relation to your pelvis.

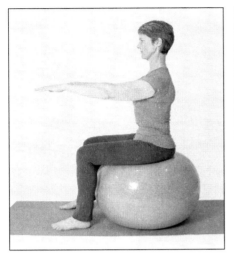

Photo 2-18

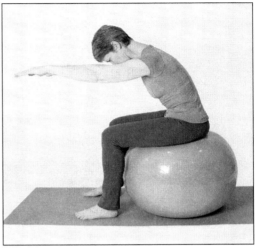

Photo 2-19

1. Sit on an exercise ball in neutral spine alignment, feet flat on the floor hip joint width apart. Raise your arms out in front of you, parallel to the floor (Photo 2-18). Avoid shrugging your shoulders.

2. On an exhale breath, round your body forward over your lap, reaching forward with your arms but keeping them parallel to the floor (Photo 2-19).

3. Inhale while you are curled over, and on the next exhale breath, starting from the base of your spine, press your spine back onto the vertical, feeling the vertebrae in your back stack on top of each other as you return to sitting upright.

4. Repeat 3 to 5 times.

Keep your weight centered over your pelvis. In this exercise you are not just leaning forward, you are rounding your body over your lap. Your weight should shift only slightly onto your feet. Feel your abdominal muscles press back against your spine, giving it a stretch. Feel lifted over your lap. Imagine there is a wall behind your body—feel your back peel away from this wall as you round forward, and feel it return to the wall as you roll back up.

Spine extension—scarecrow
This exercise activates the muscles of your upper back;
I call it the anti-computer posture exercise.

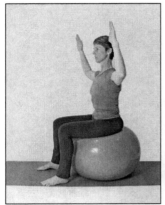 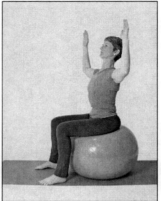 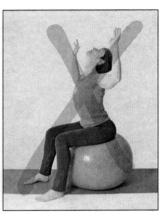

Photo 2-20   *Photo 2-21*   *Photo 2-22*

1. Sit on an exercise ball in neutral spine alignment, feet flat on the floor hip joint width apart.

2. Lift your arms out to the side with a bent elbow. Rotate your arms so that your hands reach to the ceiling—"scarecrow" position (Photo 2-20).

3. Keeping your shoulder blades wide, lift your sternum up toward the ceiling by engaging the muscles of your back between your shoulder blades (Photo 2-21). This is a small movement: think of a slight rotation of your rib cage so that your sternum barely lifts upward. Avoid taking all of the motion in your neck and low back (Photo 2-22). Keep your seat bones directly under you.

4. Hold this small thoracic extension for a few counts, and then release.

5. Repeat 3 to 5 times.

I am not particular about the breathing with this exercise, so long as you breathe!

I find it convenient and useful to combine these last two exercises. Perform one spine stretch forward and then one spine extension—scarecrow. The alternate spine flexion and spine extension enhance awareness of spine alignment. This is the sequence listed in the Suggested Workouts at the end of the book.

Plank on mat—knees

Plank is a fantastic integrating exercise for core muscle function and shoulder and leg support. Plus, it requires no equipment.

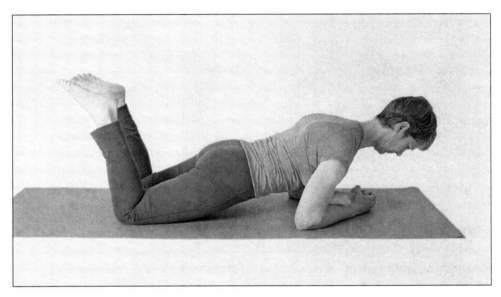

Photo 2-23

1. Lie on your stomach on a mat.

2. Bend your elbows and keep them by your sides while you place your clasped hands beneath your sternum. Bend your knees so your lower legs are off the floor.

3. While keeping your shoulders stable, lift yourself onto your knees and elbows into a suspended plank position (Photo 2-23). Seek a long and neutral spine position and avoid pulling your shoulders up around your ears. Try to keep your pelvis level and not pushed up to the ceiling.

4. Hold this position for 30 to 60 seconds.

Plank on mat—feet
A much more challenging version of the plank exercise.

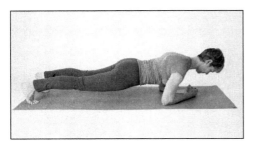

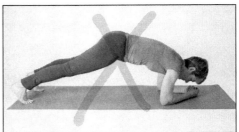

Photo 2-24   Photo 2-25

1. Lie on your stomach on a mat.

2. Bend your elbows and keep them by your sides while you place your clasped hands beneath your sternum. Keep your legs straight.

3. While keeping your shoulders stable, lift yourself onto your feet and elbows into a suspended plank position (Photo 2-24). Seek a long and neutral spine position, and avoid pulling your shoulders up around your ears. Try to keep your pelvis level and not pushed up toward the ceiling (Photo 2-25).

4. Hold this position for 30 to 60 seconds.

If plank on mat—feet is too challenging, alternate between your feet and knees for the 30 to 60 seconds of the exercise. Gradually build up the time you can hold the position on your feet. Done correctly, either plank exercise is a good integrator of abdominal and back muscles, as well as the shoulder girdle and leg muscles. When I see a rider being pulled or tossed around by her horse, I say "think plank!" to encourage body stability and balance.

Plank on ball

This exercise integrates core muscle function,
with the challenge of balance offered by the ball.

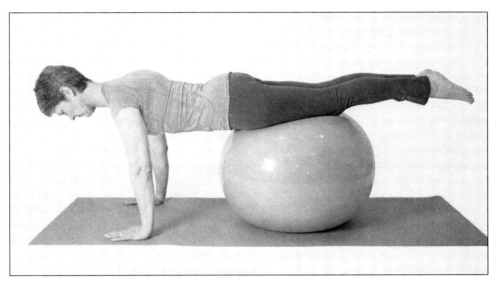

Photo 2-26

1. Lie on your stomach over an exercise ball.

2. Shift your weight toward your hands and walk your hands out onto the floor. Lift your legs up behind you so that your body is in a plank-like position, your spine in neutral alignment.

3. Begin by walking out until the front of your thighs rests on the ball (Photo 2-26). Hold this position for several breaths, then release back to lying on the ball.

4. Repeat 3 to 5 times.

Keep your abdominal muscles engaged to support your back. Keep the front of your shoulders open and your shoulder blades coming back and down, without letting your back arch.

The exercise is made more difficult by walking farther out so that the front of your knees or lower legs rest on the ball (Photo 2-27). The farther you move away from the ball, the more you will need support from your trunk muscles to maintain neutral alignment and secure balance.

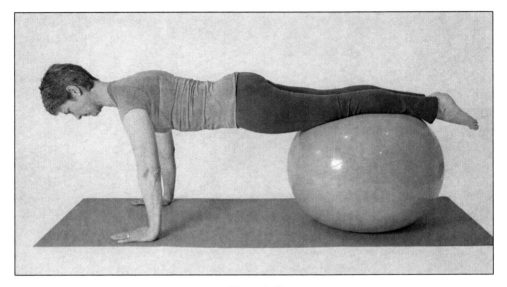

Photo 2-27

Quadruped—single

*Maintain spine position while
moving an arm or a leg.*

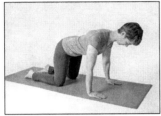 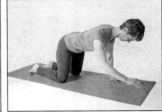 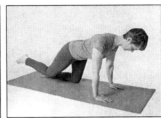

Photo 2-28   *Photo 2-29*   *Photo 2-30*

1. Start on your mat in a hands-and-knees position with knees lined up under your hip joints and hands lined up under your shoulder joints (Photo 2-28). (If this bothers your wrists, put your hands in a fist position.) Imagine your torso as a rectangular box—keep the shape of the box stable during the entire exercise.

2. On an exhale breath, extend your right arm out in front of you just far enough so it no longer supports your weight (Photo 2-29). As you inhale, bring your arm back.

3. Do the same for your left arm, right leg (slide your knee back to remove it from its support position as shown in Photo 2-30), and left leg. All the while your goal is to keep your rectangular box-like torso square.

4. Lift each arm and leg 2 to 3 times.

Quadruped—diagonal

*This more difficult version of quadruped further challenges
spine stability while you move your arms and legs.*

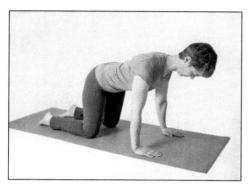

Photo 2-28

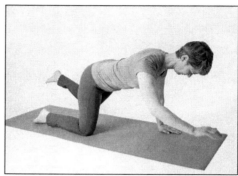

Photo 2-31

1. Start on your mat in a hands-and-knees position with knees lined up under your hip joints and hands lined up under your shoulder joints (Photo 2-28). (If this bothers your wrists, put your hands in a fist position.) Imagine your torso as a rectangular box—keep the shape of the box stable during the entire exercise.

2. On an exhale breath, extend your right arm out in front of you and your left leg out behind you at the same time (Photo 2-31). As you inhale, bring them back.

3. Repeat, extending your left arm with your right leg.

4. Lift each diagonal pair 4 to 6 times.

Avoid a large lateral shift of your weight as you lift your knee off the mat. Try to keep the center of your body stable while moving your arm and leg. This takes practice. To anchor your position, focus on your core muscles.

Abdominal Muscles: Pull In or Push Out?

I frequently encounter two questions about abdominal muscle function. The first is, "I'm told to push my abdomen or belly out in front of me. What does that mean?" And the second is, "I've been told to use my abdominals by pushing them out. How do I do that?"

The first question is simply one of semantics. A person with a rounded, flexed, or C-shaped posture may be coached to correct this posture by pushing her abdomen or belly out in front to accomplish a more upright position closer to neutral spine alignment. But to me it makes sense to address the postural issue directly and guide such a rider to use the muscles of her back to stabilize a more upright posture. I do not think the cue to "let your belly hang out in front of you" is useful, as I believe supportive tone is needed from your abdominal muscles for optimal posture and balance on a moving horse.

I teach riders to support spine stability by using the deep abdominal muscles in an inward, corset-like fashion. Many physical therapists (see Carolyn Richardson et al.) endorse this means of dynamic spine stability. It has been demonstrated that during normal spine function, the transversus abdominis (a deep abdominal muscle that creates the corset around your middle), and the multifidi (deep spine extensor muscles) are triggered to support the spine in anticipation of movement or a load. This suggests the body's innate choice for spine stability is these muscles, which work in an inward fashion. Consciously engaging these muscles facilitates dynamic spine stability and supported movement.

Other spine experts suggest that spine stability is best accomplished by bracing the abdominal muscles outward—the same way you would during a bowel movement or while giving birth. This technique of spine stability is usually recommended in the context of a brief need for spine "stiffness," such as during competitive weight lifting or delivering a karate blow to a hard surface. By pushing the abdominal muscles outward, you encase the spine in a rigid block and support the spine during the forceful movement.

Bracing the abdominal muscles outward, however, is not practical while riding for two reasons. First, this position is hard to maintain for long, and second, rigidity of the spine is not ideal while riding. There is some movement in the spine and pelvis while riding; it makes most sense to me to find a way to keep the motion within a small range by supporting this movement with the inward elastic tone of the deep abdominal and back muscles.

I personally have explored both methods of stabilizing torso position in the saddle. I find the inward corset approach logical, doable, and effective. What's more, this technique of core stability and support is what you see in any sport or activity that requires balance and movement. After all, you don't see dancers pushing out their bellies, right?

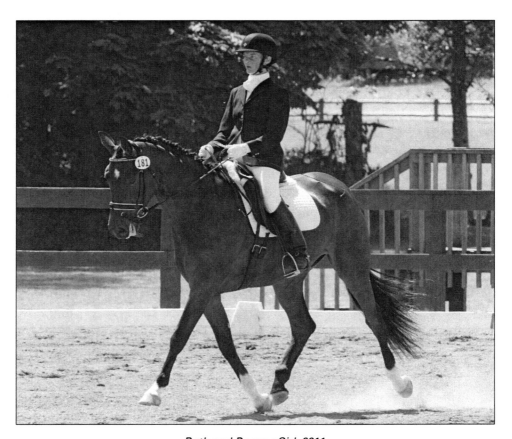

Beth and Donner Girl, 2011.

Common Posture Challenges

Many rider-position issues have at their root a problem with posture or postural support and balance.

In this book, I define ideal position in the saddle as neutral spine alignment, on the vertical. (There are circumstances, such as the forward position for jumping, where being in front of the vertical is clearly desired, but these riders should still be in neutral spine alignment.)

When first assessing any rider, I ask, "Is the rider in neutral spine alignment? If so, is the rider on the vertical, with shoulders balanced over the pelvis?" Until these criteria are met, it is very difficult to make lasting changes in any other rider position issue such as an errant arm or foot. Without the basis of stable balance from proper alignment and torso support, any adjustment of arm or leg position is likely to be fleeting.

It is not unusual to see riders who are in fairly good spine alignment but tend to ride behind the vertical, or leaning back. This position can offer some extra stability for sitting trot (see Chapter 5) but it is not the best position, as it can encourage the horse to come on its forehand. You needn't lean back to feel there is a horse in front of you! Correct spine alignment on the vertical is the best position for optimum balance in the rider—and the horse.

In addition, the position and fit of your saddle can dramatically affect your ability to find correct pelvic position and, hence, spine alignment. Get help with saddle fitting if you are fighting your saddle for correct position or are concerned about how your saddle positions your body.

Flexed, Rounded, or C-shaped Posture

Some riders tend to adopt a C-shaped alignment of the spine while in the saddle (Figure 2-10). This puts the spine in a rounded position, or spine flexion. This postural problem is not uncommon in riders who spend a great deal of their day sitting in front of a computer or desk. This posture creates problems both on and off the horse. It creates excess strain on the lower back because the body weight is pressing on the intervertebral disks in an uneven fashion. Riders with this posture often look down at their horses' necks. If they look up, as shown in Figure 2-10, this posture causes a shortened cervical spine with too much curve, and a jutting chin. This strains the disks and joints in the neck.

To correct this flexed posture, increase the activity of your back muscles to pull your upper back to a more upright position and restore the lumbar curve of your spine. This will lengthen the too-short distance between your rib cage and pelvis in the front of your body. Stretching the muscles of your shoulder girdle will also help.

If this is your posture at work, take periodic stretch breaks to disrupt this harmful position. Try the spine extension—scarecrow exercise at the computer during your workday: it does not require you to get out of your chair, it stretches and engages muscles to counteract the tendency to round forward while typing and looking at the computer screen, and it requires *no* equipment.

Take time to break this postural habit when you ride, too. This takes great focus because it is very challenging to expect your body to adopt a posture in the saddle that is different from the "norm." This flexed posture often comes packaged with overusing the gluteal (butt) muscles to aid the horse (see "The Rider's Challenge: Flexed Posture" in this chapter). These muscles can pull the pelvis into a tuck, flattening the low back. I have found that using the gluteal muscles while riding should be reserved for a few rare circumstances; many riders overuse these muscles and suffer compromised posture and hip joint mobility as a result (see Anatomy of Legs: Hip Joint Muscles in Chapter 3).

A flexed posture can be seen in a fearful rider who adopts a fetal position when the horse moves unpredictably. Unfortunately, this response is counterproductive and creates a less stable base of support and balance. Exact management of such situations must be considered individually and is beyond the scope of this discussion. However, learning good posture and postural support in and of itself can do wonders to improve your confidence in your own body and, hence, confidence in the saddle.

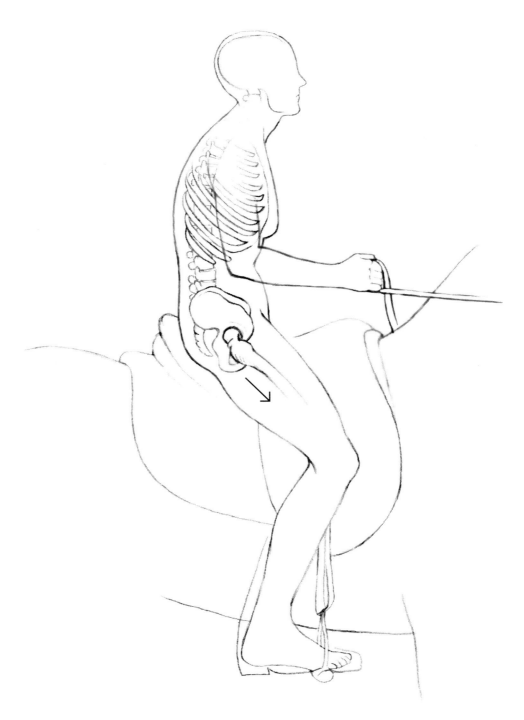

Figure 2-10. Flexed, rounded, or C-shaped posture. The seat bones point toward
the horse's shoulder (arrow), rather than straight down; the rider's shoulders
are hunched forward; and there is little or no lumbar curve in the spine.

The Rider's Challenge: Flexed Posture
Julie and Bismark

Julie asks for help with balance on her big moving Hanoverian gelding, Bismark. Despite a full-time work schedule, she manages to ride about four days a week—and she does so with great focus and commitment.

Bismark moves off in his lanky trot. His attitude is one of "I do just enough to get by." The two of them appear "earthbound," needing to work hard against gravity. In the down phase of the posting trot, Julie lands heavily behind Bismark's movement with a C-shaped posture, her legs too far in front of her. She struggles to keep Bismark in the trot and pushes him forward each time she lands in the saddle by squeezing her gluteal (butt) muscles. She sets up a cycle of kicking him forward but falling behind him in a rounded posture. Bismark carries on in a blasé manner.

Two issues contribute to Julie's difficulty keeping Bismark in an active trot: her posture, and her leg position and function. (Read more about how we resolve Julie's leg position and function problems in Chapter 3.)

Julie's flexed posture puts her center of gravity behind Bismark's and blocks him from moving forward. When she is behind his motion, her body is telling him to slow down, which she most certainly does not want. Her rounded posture makes it nearly impossible for her to come to a proper balance point in the posting trot; she is always a bit behind him.

At the halt, I have Julie do some forward and backward pelvic rocking exercises in the saddle to show how she places too much weight in the posterior (toward the tailbone) part of her pelvic floor. I move Julie's spine closer to neutral alignment by having her slightly arch her back, restoring her lumbar curve. This engages her back muscles, adjusts her pelvis so that her seat bones point downward, and releases her gluteal muscles. I have Julie make a mental note of where she feels her weight distribution over her pelvic floor. I also adjust her leg position so that her feet come back underneath her, creating the correct shoulder-hip-heel line.

Julie picks up the posting trot. Bismark is reluctant. Julie kicks harder, slipping into her C-shaped posture and falling behind his movement. Bismark, of course, slows down. I coach her to a better posture, which keeps her in balance and confers a "let's go!" attitude to her horse. Bismark responds by offering a longer stride. Julie struggles to break the habits of giving a leg aid every step, rounding her back, squeezing her gluteal muscles, and falling behind the movement. But when she keeps her spine aligned correctly and her feet underneath her, her balance improves: the two of them no longer appear earthbound, but rather in self-carriage, moving forward.

Exercises for Julie: Pelvic rocking on ball, front to back; spine extension on mat; spine extension—scarecrow; pelvic bridge—simple

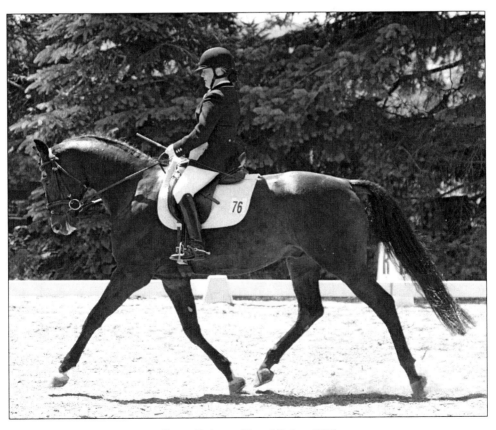

Caryn Bujnowski and Dylan, 2010.

Problems of flexed, rounded, or C-shaped posture

- Strains rider's back
- Can lead to a chair seat with rider behind the horse's movement
- Often comes packaged with rounded shoulders
- Often comes packaged with a tendency to look down
- "Closes off" the front of the rider's body, discouraging ground cover from the horse
- Invites, or is caused by, overusing the gluteal muscles
- Risks rider counterbalancing on the reins

My Challenge: Flexed Posture

I have a tendency toward a flexed, or C-shaped, posture. The function (or dysfunction) of my shoulder girdle and legs contributed to this posture. It took me some time to understand it. Sure, I got a lot of cues to "bring your shoulders back" while I was riding, but the changes I'd try to make rarely lasted because I didn't have a clear and useful tool to support better posture. It wasn't just about my arms. And, what's more, my temperament put me squarely in the "intense" category; in the saddle this translated into my focusing too much on what was happening within my line of sight instead of feeling the whole horse. So in addition to rounded shoulders and a tucked pelvis, my gaze tended downward, feeding into spine flexion.

In time I learned to use and trust my back muscles to support a correct, upright posture. Now, if I overextend my spine, my back tells me. So, I have to be careful about how much spine extension I can expect from my back. But that does not mean I don't use these muscles. Quite the contrary: improving use and awareness of my back muscles has helped me prevent back flare-ups and preserve better posture in the saddle.

Extended or Arched Posture

While many riders struggle to correct a flexed posture, an equal number ride with an extended or arched posture. Sometimes, in an effort to "sit up straight with shoulders back," a rider develops too much tone in the mid- and upper back muscles. This pulls the spine into an arch (Figure 2-11). As with Melissa (see "The Rider's Challenge: Extended Posture" in this chapter), this tension can spread to the arms and limit suppleness of the shoulder muscles, compromising contact with the horse through the bridle. This postural problem is an important cause of a "tense" or "stiff" appearance.

Using the abdominal muscles to both pull the rib cage slightly closer to the pelvis in the front of the body and lift the pubic bone up toward the sternum will correct this posture. It takes some focus to make this change; I encourage riders to feel a constant "hum" of their abdominal muscles to be sure these muscles are helping support posture. At first, many riders will feel as if they are hunched, slouched, or rounded forward. But by getting more support from the abdominal muscles, they will also feel more stable, which promotes suppleness in the shoulder girdle and a more elastic connection through the bridle. In the arched posture, the back muscles are doing most of the balance work. Accessing all of the core muscles to support posture and balance avoids straining the back muscles as the workload is spread over more muscle groups. Useful exercises include pelvic rocking on the mat or ball, and abdominal curls on the mat.

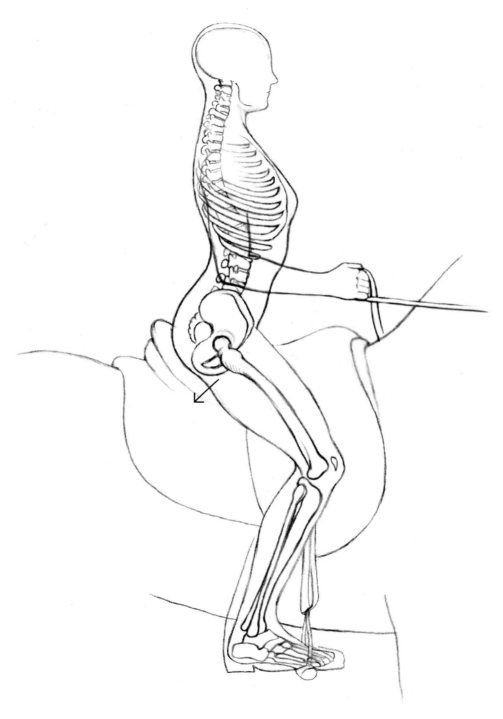

*Figure 2-11. Extended, or arched, posture. The seat bones point toward
the horse's back legs (arrow), rather than straight down; there is
too much curve in the lumbar spine; the shoulders are tight.*

The Rider's Challenge: Extended Posture
Melissa and Belle

Melissa nervously enters the arena, matching the mind-set of her 12-year-old Arab/Thoroughbred cross-mare, Belle. I ask how I might help her.

"I carry tension in my shoulders," she answers as Belle scurries off in a rapid walk.

I watch Melissa and Belle warm up at walk, trot, and canter. Melissa carries her body in a tense, upright fashion, with her shoulders living up around her ears. Her spine is arched, such that her seat bones point back toward the horse's hind feet, and her upper body tends to pitch forward. Belle trots around with quick, short steps, avoiding contact with the bit.

Melissa is correct: she carries a great deal of tension in her shoulders. Adjusting posture and increasing awareness of her center of gravity will help her improve communication with Belle.

At the halt I have Melissa do some small pelvic rocking exercises front to back in the saddle. I coach her to use her abdominal muscles, not her gluteal muscles, to move her pelvis in a tuck (this is hard to do in the saddle; it is best to first learn this movement off the horse). I have her feel how the weight underneath her pelvic floor changes toward her sacrum as her pelvis moves. I then have her stop when her seat bones are underneath her. This takes the excessive arch out of her spine, engages her abdominal muscles, and helps her feel heavier in the saddle, with positive muscle tone around her center of gravity.

"I feel like I'm hunched forward," claims Melissa.

Many with an arched posture feel slouched when their alignment is changed. I have her look in the mirror, and she sees how she looks more centered and less perched in the saddle.

"OK," she says as she views her position. "But how do I keep this position?"

I give Melissa the image of bungee cords attaching her ribs to her pelvis, preventing her spine from arching. A "hum" of tone from her abdominal muscles supports a more correct posture and eases shoulder tension.

Back out on the rail, Melissa begins to revert to her arched position.

I coach her to keep the bungee cords short to keep her ribs down, and to feel the weight over her pelvic floor shift back toward her sacrum.

At the posting trot Melissa begins to feel a more stable balance. However, when Belle speeds up, Melissa reverts to her arched posture and tense shoulders and pulls on the reins. I coach her to steady Belle's trot tempo with her posting tempo, and to breathe and focus on her core for balance to decrease tension in her shoulders.

Belle begins to respond to Melissa's improved posture and balance by keeping a steadier trot tempo. For some steps Belle even begins to lower her head and reach to the bit.

Exercises for Melissa: Pelvic rocking on ball, front to back; abdominal curls; bounce in rhythm 2—arm swings; spine stretch forward

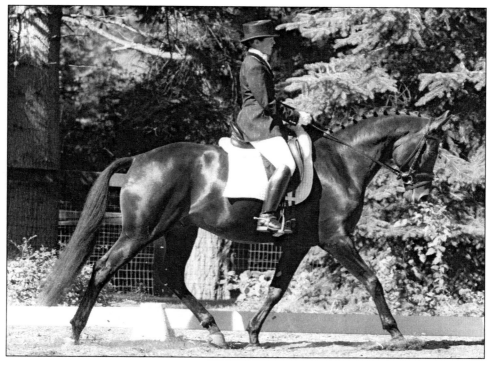

Catherine Reid and Eisenherz (owned by Kathie Vigoroux and Sherry Tourino), 2010.

Problems with extended or arched posture
- Causes rider to appear tense and feel unstable
- Limits suppleness in the shoulder girdle
- Makes it hard to find elastic contact
- Pulls rider's focus up and away from center of gravity
- Encourages riding from shoulders and hands, not from the center of the body
- Creates precarious balance
- Causes low or mid back pain from overuse and poor posture
- Perches rider on top of the horse, not sitting and moving with the horse

---

S-shaped Posture

Some riders, especially those with a long and tall torso, ride with too much curve in the lumbar, thoracic, and cervical regions of the spine. The back is overarched in the lumbar region, and the pelvis is tilted such that the seat bones point back. At the same time, the rider's upper back is rounded and behind the vertical, while the shoulders are rounded forward. There may also be too much curve in the neck such that the chin juts forward (Figure 2-12 A). The long torso is challenging to support and keep stable on horseback. For these riders, the problem often starts with their tendency to position the upper body behind the vertical with shoulders rounded forward. The other regions of the spine, the low back and the neck, compensate for this off-balanced position with increased curvature.

These riders often find it difficult to ride comfortably, and some complain of back pain. These riders often look unstable and too moveable in their midsection, as their postural support is unsteady and unbalanced. The forward-positioned chin and tight shoulders can cause a head bob, particularly noticeable at sitting trot. It is very challenging to address all of the regions of the spine at once, but without doing so, stability and balance is precarious.

For this postural issue, I first adjust the pelvis so that the seat bones point down. This requires abdominal muscle activation, bringing the pubic bone of the pelvis closer to the sternum of the rib cage. However, if that is the only correction, the rider remains rounded forward in the upper back

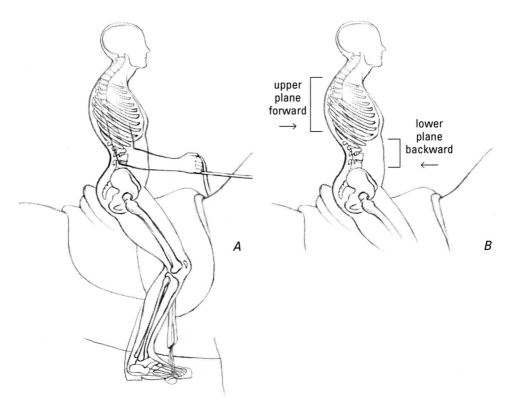

upper
plane
forward
→

lower
plane
backward
←

A

B

*Figure 2-12. A. S-shaped posture or overly curved spine. There is excessive
lumbar curve; the upper back is behind the vertical with excessive curve in the
thoracic spine (where the ribs attach). This results in a forward-thrusting
head with too much curve in the cervical spine.
B. Feel a plane of the upper back and a plane in the lower abdomen;
when these planes come toward the middle of the body, excess curves
are removed and the spine is supported in better alignment.*

and shoulders, with continued stress at the neck. So, at the same time as activating the abdominal muscles, the upper back muscles must also engage to bring the thoracic spine into a straighter alignment, lift the sternum, and bring the shoulders back and down. Finally, to straighten the cervical spine, the rider needs to stretch upward through the back of the neck, as if "on the bit." To help hold the position in the body, I suggest that riders imagine that the upper back is one plane, and the abdominal region is another plane. These two planes are parallel to each other but are separated by the width of the rider's body. To achieve improved spine alignment and stability, both planes are drawn toward the center of the body (Figure 2-12 B). This dynamic activity lengthens the spine and takes the excess curvature out of the lumbar and thoracic spines. The neck position then often corrects itself or is relatively easy to reposition.

The plank on ball and plank on mat exercises, done correctly, will strengthen the muscles that pull the two body planes together in the middle. However, it is easy to perform these exercises incorrectly and exaggerate the excess curves. Prepare carefully for these exercises and think "shoulders back and down, and abdominal muscles inward" at the same time. If this results in pain or straining, stop and seek input. The exercise spine extension—scarecrow also facilitates support of the thoracic spine.

The Rider's Challenge: S-shaped Posture
Jennifer and Jupiter

Jennifer, an experienced and advanced rider, contacts me for a position consultation.

"I dislike watching my videotapes from the horse shows. I don't like the lack of elegance in my position. Plus, my back is sometimes sore after riding," she explains.

Jennifer rides a 5-year-old Thoroughbred/Percheron-cross gelding, Jupiter. Jennifer is a positive leader for the young horse, but he tends to be heavy on his forehand, barreling around the arena.

I watch Jennifer as she rides Jupiter in a forward posting trot, sitting trot, and canter. Jennifer has a slight build, long legs, and a long torso. It is challenging to maintain this long spine in a stable neutral position, especially in the context of a heavy horse. Jupiter's balance difficulties have affected Jennifer's posture and effectiveness: she has adopted a classic S-shaped position that has her upper body rounded back behind the vertical, with too much arch in her lumbar spine. Further, to counterbalance her backward-leaning upper body, her chin juts out. The backward leaning and rounded upper body is likely in response to Jupiter's being on the forehand: Jennifer uses her body weight against his leaning, supporting a mutual "hold each other up" situation. The resulting tightness of her shoulder girdle causes a head bob visible in the sitting trot. As well, excessive lumbar spine movement makes her appear unstable in the sitting trot, rather than elegant and balanced. This excess movement of the lumbar spine could be causing her back soreness.

At the halt, I give Jennifer my "planes" images: I have her imagine that the back of her upper body forms one plane. The front of her lower body, or her abdominal region, forms another plane. To promote stability of her long torso, I have her picture the two planes coming close together in the middle of her body. This activates the spine extensors in her upper back to support a more upright, less-rounded upper back position, as well as the abdominal muscles, to support a less-arched lumbar spine. As a final cue, I have her stretch the back of her neck long, imagining that she is "on the bit." These three maneuvers take out the excessive curves in her lumbar, thoracic, and cervical spine regions, and activate postural muscles to preserve this alignment despite Jupiter's pulling. To test her ability to keep this alignment, I stand in front of Jupiter's chest, hold onto to the reins, and pull against Jennifer's body and posture. By keeping her planes coming together in the middle of her body, she maintains proper posture despite the load.

Jennifer struggles to preserve this new alignment in sitting trot. I encourage Jennifer to do circles or transitions to help Jupiter's balance, rather than slip into her usual holding pattern. With improved awareness of how Jupiter coaxes her into holding him up, she becomes more particular about him maintaining his own balance, and rides with improved precision and higher standards.

Jennifer's sliding into her S posture demonstrates how horses can change us! Setting high posture and alignment standards for ourselves makes us better horse trainers: in a position of clear and stable balance, we can more readily detect and correct the horse's problem.

Exercises for Jennifer: Pelvic rocking supine, spine extension—scarecrow, plank on ball, plank on mat—knees and feet

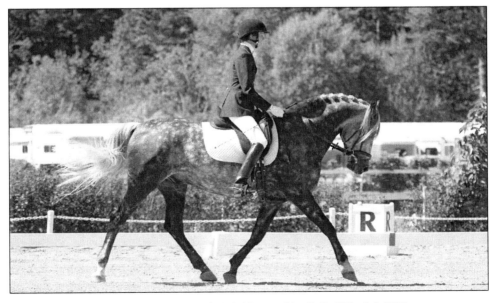

Garyn Heideman and Gabriel (owned by Kelly O'Toole), 2010.

Problems with S-shaped posture
- Causes unstable balance
- Puts rider behind the motion, "leaning" on the reins
- Extends lumbar spine, leaving it unsupported and risking strain
- Extends cervical spine, leaving it unsupported and risking strain
- Leads to a head bob due to the associated tight shoulder girdle
- Precludes self-carriage in both horse and rider as they are "holding each other up" through the bridle

Lateral Postural Imbalance

Imbalance of the postural muscles can interfere with side-to-side, or lateral, symmetry. I am amazed at how often this type of imbalance occurs in riders. I have seen it in more than half of the riders I have worked with, from beginning to advanced. Positive changes in rider lateral balance can bring remarkable improvements in horse and rider function, balance, and harmony.

Seemingly small adjustments in how you support your body can improve your horse's way of going and response to aids. It is a rider position issue, more than any other, where your horse's way of going gives you immediate feedback. The horse's improvement quickly informs you that you've made positive changes in your position, even though they are difficult, argue with habits, and do not feel normal!

Consequences of lateral postural imbalance
- Makes straightness of the horse very difficult
- Risks giving horse conflicting aids
- Makes balance in bending lines and lateral movements very difficult
- Creates or contributes to lateral imbalance in the horse

No one is perfectly symmetric, and, just like our horses, most of us have a tendency to be stronger on one side than the other. The muscles on the strong side of the body are shorter and will tend to pull the pelvis and thighbone up off the saddle, causing an inward curve of that side of the body. This shifts weight onto the pelvis and seat bone of the weaker, longer side (Figure 2-13 B). This is usually accompanied by a slight spinal rotation toward the stronger side. Often, but not always, this asymmetry is related to handedness; that is, a right-handed rider will tend to have a stronger right side of the body. The right side is shorter, weight is shifted onto the left seat bone, and the right arm and leg are dominant. While we might overcome and correct these imbalances during daily activities without much problem, they become much more pronounced in the precarious and unpredictable environment of riding.

This right-to-left asymmetry is sometimes described as "collapsing," that is, the rider is collapsing on the short, strong side. In some ways it looks like the rider is falling over toward the short side. This is not the best way to describe the problem, however, as collapsing implies being passive or soft. This imbalance is anything but passive or soft. The short side is the overactive and strong side; the long, weighted side is the side that is not doing its part to support position, symmetry, and balance.

Sometimes an instructor might guide a rider to "push weight onto" or "sit down on" the lifted side of the pelvis or seat bone. But, since muscles only shorten and pull to move bones, there is no way to push the lifted seat bone down onto the saddle. This asymmetry is best corrected by thinking of engaging the trunk muscles of the longer, weaker side and lifting weight off the heavily weighted side of the pelvis. This leads to a more balanced use of the muscles of the sides of the trunk and equalizes the weight distribution over the seat bones and pelvic floor in the saddle (Figure 2-13 A). It takes great energy and focus to change this habitual support pattern. Improving lateral balance starts with awareness and muscle coordination. The following exercises help develop awareness and symmetry in the trunk muscles.

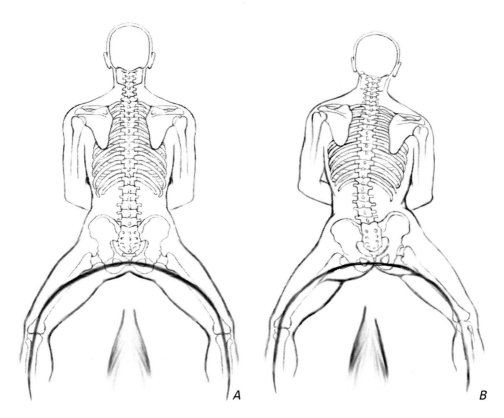

Figure 2-13. A. The rider on the left has good lateral balance.
B. The rider on the right shows a lateral imbalance: the right side is shortened;
the weight is shifted to the left; and the right shoulder is low, the left shoulder is high.
This is often accompanied by a pulling up and in of the right hip joint muscles,
and losing the stirrup on this short side.

Pelvic rocking on ball, side to side
*Use your back and abdominal muscles to adjust
the lateral position of the pelvis.*

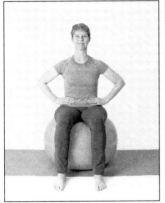 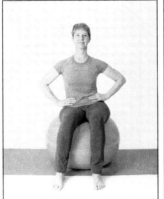 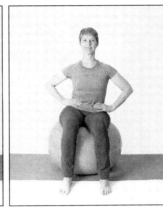

Photo 2-32   *Photo 2-33*   *Photo 2-34*

1. Sit on an exercise ball in neutral alignment, feet in front of you, flat on the floor, hip-joint-width apart.

2. Place your hands on your waist: this helps you feel the trunk muscles engage during the exercise (Photo 2-32).

3. Lift up the left side of your pelvis, engaging the trunk muscles on that side, while sinking weight onto your right seat bone (Photo 2-33). Imagine that you are shortening the distance between your armpit and pelvis on your left side.

4. Come back to start position, and repeat on your right side (Photo 2-34).

5. Do 8 to 10 swings side to side.

Most have one side for which this exercise is straightforward (the strong side), and one side for which it is not (the weaker side). Feel what happens on the strong or straightforward side. Try to duplicate on the weaker side.

Be careful not to shift your shoulders to the side or twist your body. The motion is a small side-to-side movement of your pelvis by the trunk muscles, like a swinging pendulum. Try not to use your gluteal muscles or other leg muscles to move your pelvis. Keep your feet flat on the floor.

Spine twist on ball
*Spine twist improves awareness of
lateral balance while turning.*

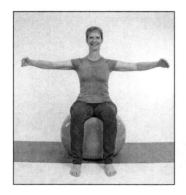 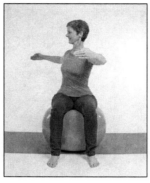 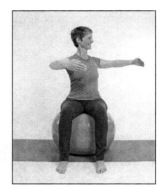

Photo 2-35   *Photo 2-36*   *Photo 2-37*

1. Sit upright on an exercise ball, feet on the floor, hip joint width apart.

2. Lift up your arms and hold them in a big circle out in front of you, as if you were holding a huge ball (Photo 2-35).

3. Take an easy inhale breath, and on the exhale breath, rotate your upper body (rib cage, shoulders, and head) to the right (Photo 2-36). Then inhale back to center and exhale while you rotate your upper body to the left (Photo 2-37) and inhale back to center.

4. Repeat this twist or rotation of your spine 6 to 8 times each direction.

Keep your seat bones equally weighted during this exercise. It is tempting to sink onto your seat bone on the side opposite the direction of the twist (Photo 2-38). If you do find yourself sinking, keep that seat bone lifted so that your weight stays in the middle of the ball throughout the movement (using the tools taught above in pelvic rocking on ball, side to side). Keep your upper body moving as one unit, so your arms do not move more than your torso. Let your gaze follow the movement.

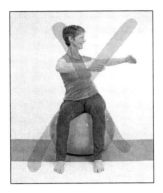

Photo 2-38

This exercise helps you learn that you can move your upper body independently from your lower body, and that you can turn your upper body without an obligatory shift in weight. This allows you, while riding your horse on a circle, to keep your shoulders in line with your horse's shoulders and at the same time keep your weight balanced over your horse's back.

Side planks—knees
*Side planks strengthen the muscles in your waist,
developing a tool for lateral balance.*

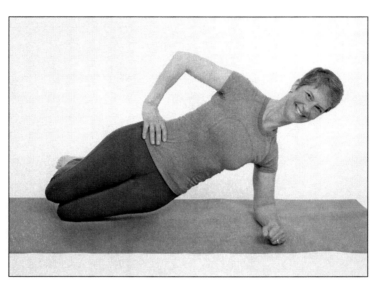

Photo 2-39

1. Lie on your left side with your left elbow in line under your left armpit; your upper arm bone should be perpendicular to the floor.

2. Stack one leg on top of the other, positioned so that they are in line with the rest of your body, with your hip joints straight. Bend your knees so the lower legs are behind you.

3. Place your right hand on your waist.

4. From the muscles of your left waist, lift yourself up onto your left elbow and your left knee by engaging the core muscles of your left torso (Photo 2-39). Keep your body lifted from the middle, as if a rope were around your midsection pulling you up to the ceiling.

5. Hold the position for 15 to 30 seconds.

6. Repeat on the right side.

Be careful that you do not push away from your elbow; your upper arm should stay perpendicular to the floor. Too much angle at the shoulder is straining.

Side planks—feet
A much more challenging version of side planks.

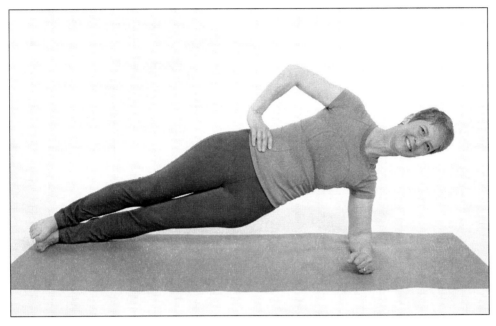

Photo 2-40

1. Lie on your left side, with your left elbow in line under your left armpit.

2. Stack one leg on top of the other, positioned so that they are in line with the rest of your body with your knee and hip joints straight.

3. Place your right hand on your waist.

4. From the muscles of your left waist, lift yourself up onto your left elbow and your left foot by engaging the core muscles of your left torso (Photo 2-40). If this is too challenging, place one foot in front of the other. Keep your body lifted from the middle, as if a rope were around your mid-section pulling you up to the ceiling.

5. Hold the position for 15 to 30 seconds.

6. Repeat on the right side.

Be careful that you do not push away from your elbow; your upper arm should stay perpendicular to the floor. Too much angle at the shoulder is straining.

The Rider's Challenge: Lateral Balance
Christina and Max

Christina trots up on her attractive, grey Oldenburg gelding, Max. She is smartly turned out and quite earnest in her attitude.

"I need for him to be more responsive to my aids," she says.

I watch the two of them for a few minutes. Christina has a fairly short torso with proper spine alignment front to back. As she executes a right turn at the posting trot, however, she falls off to the left and overbends Max's neck to the right. He resists and tosses his head; Christina responds by more pulling on the right rein and a kick with her right leg. They continue around the right turn with Max in a flat, irregular trot rhythm, resisting the right rein and falling to the left.

On the left rein, Christina turns her body to the right and crosses her right (outside) hand over Max's neck to the left to get Max to turn left. He resists and tosses his counterbent neck, his trot again losing a regular rhythm.

Christina's lateral balance is contributing to the communication difficulties with Max. She is short and contracted on her right side, with her weight shifted to the left, regardless of direction of travel.

I have Christina do the pelvic rocking side to side and spine twist exercises in the saddle to help her become aware of her unbalanced weight distribution over her pelvic floor. It is very difficult for her to accomplish lifting the left side of her pelvis with the muscles of her left waist region, and she resorts to lifting her left shoulder, twisting her body, and lifting her left leg. With some persistence, she is able to connect to the muscles of her left torso and improve her balance over her pelvic floor.

I point out that just like our horses, our bodies have their own "evasions" and assure Christina that she is not alone with this balance challenge. Day-to-day living results in right-left asymmetries in our body. When we put ourselves in the precarious and unpredictable position of being on horseback, these habits come in loud and strong. It takes a huge conscious effort to change them. Correcting this asymmetry starts with awareness. Then we try to replace the engrained habits with more productive stabilizing strategies. Our horses quickly reward us when our alignment improves.

I have Christina track left and think of her body bending left in the same way she wants her horse to bend left. By rotating her upper body to the left and engaging her left waist, Christina keeps her shoulders aligned with Max's shoulders and reduces her excessive weight on her left seat bone. It is difficult for her to make these changes, but each time she convinces her body to rotate left and be more centered, she is able to release her overly tight grip on the right (outside) rein, and Max's neck stretches toward the bit and his trot gains cadence.

"I can't believe the change in his trot with what feels like such a tiny change in my body!" she exclaims.

To the right, Christina has a much more difficult time accessing the left side of her body to keep herself in lateral balance. She persists in over-rotating her body to the right and hanging on the right rein while the two of them fall to the left.

I have Christina rotate her upper body a bit left, or to the outside, to correct her excessive rightward rotation. I have her think of steering Max's shoulders: to turn him right, bring his left shoulder to the right. I have her lift her weight off her left pelvis to bring Max to the right, by engaging the muscles of her left waist. Two images help her: a rope around her waist pulling her to the center of the circle (activating her left waist muscles) and bringing her left side to the right, and installing a "spur" on her left elbow that prevents her body from slopping too far left.

Christina struggles with her balance to the right, but when she is able to shift her weight from off the left seat bone onto the middle of her pelvis, she becomes more elastic in the contact through the right rein, Max is straighter, and again, he reaches for the bit with improved cadence.

"My brain is exhausted," she says at the end of the ride. "But Max was better!"

This lateral balance issue is such a challenge to work on because our movement habits can be very engrained. Max rewarded Christina for her efforts—there is no better feedback than that!

Exercises for Christina: Pelvic rocking on ball, side to side; spine twist on ball, side planks—knees and feet

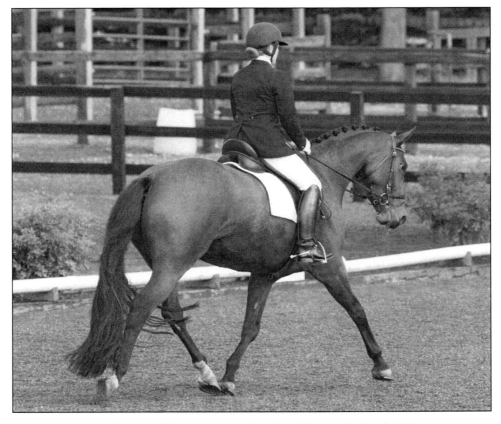

Lisa Boyer and Zamora (owned by Dutch Equine Stables), 2010.

Lateral imbalances affect horse and rider function in both overt and subtle ways. These are some manifestations of lateral imbalance that I have observed (a given rider may have one or more). Note to instructors: To get more information about the horse and rider's lateral balance, stand and watch from outside the circle, rather than from the middle of the circle.

The "right-sided" rider:
- Sits too far to the left tracking to the right, causing the horse to fall out the left shoulder.
- Sits to the left tracking left, so the horse resists left bend or falls in on the circle left.
- Rotates her upper body to the right tracking both to the right and to the left.
- Tends to overuse the right arm and rein regardless of direction of travel; the horse's neck is overbent going to the right; the horse's

neck is restricted and either counterbent or not allowed to bend left when tracking left.

- Tightens her right leg, with the right knee pulled up and into the knee roll of the saddle. The right leg has to grip to prevent her from falling farther off to the left side. As a result, the rider tends to lose the right stirrup and has a hard time controlling the right leg.
- Heavily weights the left stirrup, sometimes pressing the leg forward. The left leg may lack function because it is stuck carrying excess weight.
- Has a right shoulder that is lower than the left shoulder.
- Tilts head to the right.

The "left-sided" rider:

- Sits too far to the right tracking to the left, causing the horse to fall out the right shoulder.
- Sits to the right tracking right, so the horse resists right bend or falls in on the circle right.
- Rotates her upper body to the left tracking both to the right and to the left.
- Tends to overuse the left arm and rein regardless of direction of travel; the horse's neck is overbent going to the left; the horse's neck is restricted and either counterbent or not allowed to bend right when tracking right.
- Tightens her left leg, with the left knee pulled up and into the knee roll of the saddle. The left leg has to grip to prevent her from falling farther off to the right side. As a result, the rider tends to lose the left stirrup and has a hard time controlling the function of the left leg.
- Heavily weights the right stirrup, sometimes pressing the leg forward. The right leg may lack function because it is stuck carrying excess weight.
- Has a left shoulder that is lower than the right shoulder.
- Tilts head to the left.

Lateral imbalance can complicate lateral movements. For example, the leg yield can be quite different depending upon direction.

For a right-sided rider, the leg yield may be relatively easy going to the left because the rider already sits in that direction. Balance during the left leg yield, however, may not be good because the horse might tend to fall onto the leading left shoulder. The leg yield to the right can be challenging because the rider's weight is to the left but the aids are trying say "go to the right." This can lead to confusion and resistance in the horse and the "need" for stronger and stronger aids from the rider. Vice versa for a left-sided rider.

Lateral balance habits can make a simple problem worse. Imagine a right-sided rider sitting left while tracking right, and the horse is falling out the left shoulder. The rider may respond by adding more inside rein, which will overbend the horse's neck, causing the horse to fall even more to the left. The unsuspecting rider reacts by pulling more on the right rein, further activating her right side and shifting her weight farther to the left; the horse falls more out the left shoulder and farther away from the desired direction of travel. This unbalanced picture can be dysfunctional enough to disturb the horse's rhythm or send the pair into the arena wall.

On a circle to the left, a right-sided rider tends to sit with weight shifted to the left, or to the inside of a circle. Her body is also rotated to the right, so her shoulders are not aligned with the horse's shoulders. On a left circle, the horse tends to fall in on the left shoulder. The rider may try to "hold up" the horse's left shoulder either with the left (inside) rein or may try to rebalance through the right (outside) rein. The right rein may already be restricted by the rider's dominant right side and arm. This further unbalances the horse onto the left shoulder and gives the horse a mixed message ("go left" with the left rein; "don't go left" with the right rein). It is hard for the rider to access her left leg to encourage left bend as her balance is unsteady, her left leg is heavily weighted, and the left leg and side tend to be the lazy side anyway.

Doing simple ball exercises in the saddle can improve lateral symmetry. Pelvic rocking side to side in the saddle will help you access the torso muscles on the long, less-strong side of your body and introduce the feeling of being truly in the middle of the saddle. Again, the pelvic floor reference is helpful to guide you to feel that it is possible to keep fairly even weight over both right and left seat bones when your pelvis is centered in the saddle from balanced torso muscle function. When practicing this exercise in the saddle, however, be sure to use the muscles of your torso, not the muscles of your legs (particularly your gluteal muscles and/or your hip flexors), to adjust pelvic position. If your leg muscles move your pelvis, they become involved in posture and postural support and are not available for leg aids. It is very important for you to make adjustments in your posture or pelvic position using your torso muscles.

The spine twist exercise, done in a small range of motion, teaches you that it is possible to turn your upper body a little bit in both directions without disturbing the weight over your pelvic floor. You learn the skill of turning your upper body either right or left and are thus able to keep your shoulders aligned with your horse's shoulders, regardless of direction of travel and without disturbing balance.

If you struggle with lateral balance, you may find it helpful to imagine a small spur (like the one you may wear on your boot) on the inside of the elbow of your long, heavily weighted side. The job of this "elbow spur" is to keep the long side tucked in and engaged, doing its part to help stabilize alignment and balance.

Imagine you are a right-sided rider. When tracking right, you need to prevent your weight from falling too far to the left. Your left "elbow spur" keeps your torso going a bit to the right and prevents it from bowing out to the left. It may help to think of steering your horse's withers by bringing the left side of your body toward the right. This helps keep weight appropriately on your right seat bone. You must be careful to not overbend the horse's neck to accomplish the turn; instead, bring the outside of your horse to the right with your torso and, sometimes, with your left upper thigh.

When tracking left, you must make a conscious effort to turn your shoulders to the left and rotate your body a bit to the left; in essence, you, like your horse, need to bend left. This is not a natural way of positioning yourself, but in doing so, your weight will be more centered, and your left leg will be able to support your horse's bend. Rotating your torso left with the horse's shoulders also guides you to allow the left bend of the horse's neck through the right (outside) rein. Your left "elbow spur" keeps up its job of activating your left torso, as well.

When you achieve improved balance going right and then left, changes of direction can be introduced through, for example, a figure of eight. This movement helps you hone in on finding and staying in the middle of the saddle regardless of direction of travel. With improved balance, your horse's way of going will dramatically improve, and the resistances and evasions will lessen.

My recommendations for where to place your weight while turning may differ from other instructors' advice. Some advocate sitting heavy on the inside seat bone (that is, shifting weight to the right while tracking right). I must respectfully disagree with this guide and encourage you to stay in the middle of the saddle regardless of direction. Rather than overtly shifting weight, send your energy or center in the direction of travel. Trying to weight one seat bone more than the other risks your getting crooked and twisted. It is hard enough to stay in the middle of the saddle. But from this position, you gain better function of all of your aids—center, legs, and arms. Rider and horse balance is optimized.

Certainly the horse's balance and asymmetries play a role in the scenarios I've described, but since you are the cognitive, problem-solving member of the partnership, you must recognize your role in this lateral (or any other!) balance problem. When you have found stability and balance in the middle of the saddle, you can then influence your horse and help it balance more efficiently. You are able to quickly feel if your horse falls one way or the other and can help your horse regain balance, rather than make it worse. You become more perceptive and effective.

> **Since you are the cognitive, problem-solving member of the partnership, you must recognize your role in this lateral (or any other!) balance problem.**

Lateral postural imbalances are hard to address when your front-to-back balance is unstable. When I train riders, I do not focus on lateral balance until there is an understanding of the balance between the muscles of the front and the back of the body.

Lateral asymmetry can get worse when working on a new movement or figure. The effort devoted to learning the new material prompts the brain to return to its habitual balance patterns. The need for strong arm or leg aids can also challenge your stability to the point that this postural imbalance becomes more pronounced. As in horse training, I advise riders to take a step back when the balance gets worse, correct it, regroup, and try again. And don't forget to breathe!

Unbalanced X Posture

A final postural problem, the unbalanced X posture, is very challenging to address. It is one where the rider has a more complicated asymmetry that causes her weight at the pelvis to go one direction and her upper body to go the other. Straightness for the horse is thus very challenging.

Imagine your torso as a rectangle. Draw a line from your right shoulder to your left pelvis, and your left shoulder to your right pelvis. You have drawn an X on your torso. Most people have equal arms of this X. Some, however, particularly those with scoliosis, or abnormal lateral curvature of the spine, have one arm of the X longer than the other (Figure 2-14). At times I have

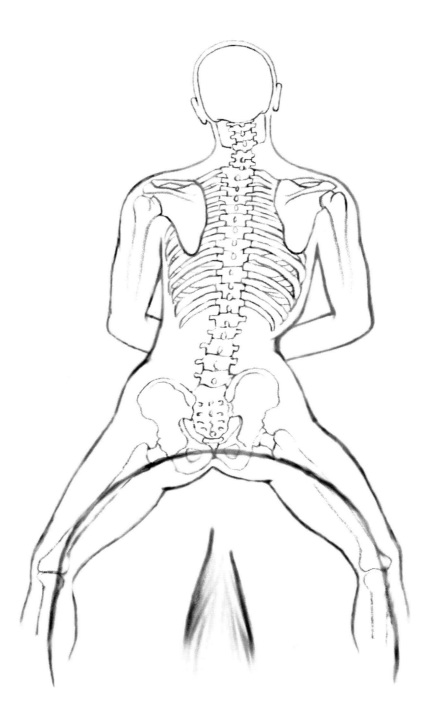

Figure 2-14. Unbalanced X posture. The distance between the right shoulder and
left pelvis is longer than the distance between the left shoulder and right pelvis. This
imbalance can be corrected by imagining a plane under the right armpit pressing to the
center of the body, and a plane at the left pelvis pressing to the center of the body.

seen this compensation in riders with a lateral imbalance problem. Rather than truly addressing the unbalanced weight over both seat bones, the crafty body of some riders will adjust by simply shifting the mobile upper body and shoulders to the less-weighted side of the body. The pelvis remains too far off to one side, with the shoulders too far to the other. This takes one problem and creates two!

This is a challenging balance strategy to correct, particularly if an underlying spinal rotation exists. But, if you have this issue, you can begin to feel straighter with an exercise. Let's say that your X imbalance has your right-shoulder-to-left-pelvis distance longer than your left-shoulder-to-right-pelvis distance. To be straight, you need to shift your rib cage to the left and shift your pelvis to the right. You can begin to feel this by putting your right hand under your right armpit and pressing to the center of your body. At the same time, put your left hand on the left side of your pelvis and press it toward the center of your body. These movements bring the two arms of your torso "X" closer to symmetry. Your torso becomes more like a rectangle than a slanted parallelogram. As well, keeping your elbows close by the sides of your rib cage can help you recognize when your rib cage tends to shift to one side or the other—your arms define a corridor for your body. Other helpful exercises include pelvic rocking on ball, side to side; spine twist on ball; plank on mat—knees and feet; plank on ball; side planks—knees and feet; and quadruped.

Riders, Keep Your Backs Healthy!

It is estimated that more than 80 percent of Americans will at some point in their lives experience back pain severe enough to interfere with work and quality of life. The incidence in horseback riders is not known but is likely at least as high, given the nature of the sport.

Horseback riding can contribute to back pain if good posture and body mechanics are not maintained. Riding-specific recommendations for preserving back health are covered in this book. Basically, keep correct posture in the saddle!

Also consider the lifting and schlepping associated with horse care—much of it can be very back unfriendly. Pay attention to body alignment and mechanics during barn chores. Avoid twisting while lifting. Keep proper spine alignment while carrying heavy objects, and lift objects by bending your legs, not your spine. A good rule of thumb is to keep "your nose aligned with your toes" to prevent twisting and back strain. Move your feet to fork manure into the wheelbarrow; avoid rotating your torso. Keep heavy objects close to the front of your body. Keep focused on the task at hand so body and mind work together. Split heavy loads into several lighter loads or get help. Use a tractor or wheelbarrow whenever possible. Use a step stool to groom a large horse so you needn't reach and twist to get at his back. Avoid fatigue! Just as with horses, this is when injuries are likely to occur.

Carefully consider the type of horse you ride. If you have back troubles, weigh the risks and benefits of working with a very green horse: the inevitable sudden movements are not ideal for your vulnerable back (while riding, leading, or lunging). Also consider the conformation of your horse. A horse with a very round barrel may force your thighbone into a position that causes back strain. A large horse requires more lifting and reaching while grooming and tacking up. Work to improve the quality of your horse's trot before trying to sit it if it is jarring.

Barn setup can facilitate back-friendly horse care. Frequent hose bibs and hoses minimize the need to carry water. A hayloft allows

gravity to deliver hay rather than your lifting it. Be sure walking sur-
faces are not slippery to minimize the risk of falls. Use a tractor that
fits you to avoid reaching and straining for foot pedals and gearshifts.
Make sure your horse trailer is equipped with an easily lifted ramp or
a step up, and consider a motorized jack for hookup.

It may seem obvious, but remember to take good care of your
body. Back health is supported by good nutrition and fitness. A good
fitness program includes a mix of aerobic activity, as well as core,
arm, and leg strengthening and stretching.

Finally, listen to your body. Do not ignore aches and pains. It is
cheaper to hire help than to destroy your back (remember, you only
have one). Depending upon your back problem, horse riding and
horse care may be doable, but you must respect your body.

Seeking and maintaining proper posture improves your awareness of your horse's imbalances. Fine-tuning your balance helps you quickly recognize when your horse's issues threaten to change your body position. Allowing your horse's movement and evasions to change your posture makes you a less effective rider. Defining and maintaining correct posture makes you a clear leader, able to set precise standards for you and your horse.

With a secure posture, the goals of body control—awareness and control of your legs and arms—become much more reasonable and doable. Next we'll talk about these body parts.

CHAPTER 3

Control Your Body: Legs

Effective riding requires control of your legs and arms. Control of your legs and arms can only come from a balanced position in the saddle. Chapter 2 emphasizes the importance of basing balance in the torso. Without this tool, the body seeks balance from the arms and/or legs, creating unnecessary and unwanted tension. This precludes having independent, efficient, and effective aids.

Control of your legs and arms can only come from a balanced position in the saddle.

Without awareness and control, your legs fall into the role of "muscle men," causing you to use force to get what you want. You need to feel as if your legs are part of your horse's body (Figure 3-1). Your legs must move with your horse's swinging

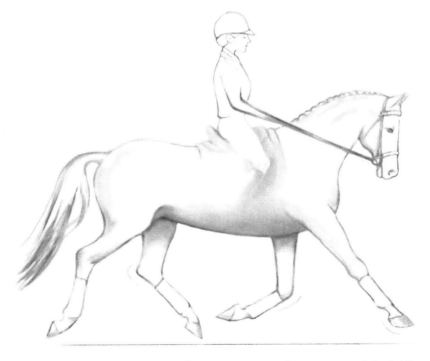

Figure 3-1. Riding in balance allows your arms to become part of the bridle and your legs to become part of your horse's body.

barrel or rib cage, and give appropriately timed aids to ask for more activity, engagement, or a lateral step. You must have suitable control so you can use your right leg, left leg, or both for an aid. More advanced control allows you to use different parts of your leg for different purposes. Giving leg aids must not disrupt your balance or impair your horse's movement. A leg that is gripping to keep you from falling off cannot move with or aid your horse effectively. But you can only release a gripping leg when you do not need it for security—that is, when your balance is centered in your torso.

By design, in this chapter I give basic descriptions of various leg muscle functions. It is impossible to sort out, during the busy act of riding, precisely which muscle does what when. When I say, for example, "Don't use your gluteal muscles," that really means use them *less*. It is not possible to have any single muscle group do nothing. My examples and illustrations show extremes to make the problems obvious. It is common for a rider to have more than one issue. But as you become aware, you can address problems and improve your effectiveness with balanced and supple leg muscle function.

Anatomy of Legs: Bones

The leg connects to the pelvis at the hip joint (Figure 3-2) and is held in place with multiple strong ligaments. The hip joint is a "ball and socket" joint, which makes a great range and variety of motion possible. The thighbone (femur) can move forward in flexion, a bit back in extension (the hip joint does not have a big range of motion in extension), out to the side in abduction, toward the center of the body in adduction, or inward (internal) or outward (external) rotation. It is a joint that is meant to move.

The knee joint (Figure 3-2) is essentially a hinge joint and moves primarily in two dimensions: flexion, or bending the knee, and extension, or straightening the knee. This joint is not able to allow rotation or abduction/adduction (outward/inward motion) of the lower leg to any significant degree. This will become important when we talk about how to apply leg aids.

The ankle joint is a complex joint that allows movement of the foot upward in flexion or downward in extension (or pointing the toe, also called dorsiflexion); the foot can also rotate inward (inversion or rolling onto the baby toe) and outward (eversion or rolling onto the great toe). Keeping the muscles of this joint supple and not locked allows the ankle to absorb movement.

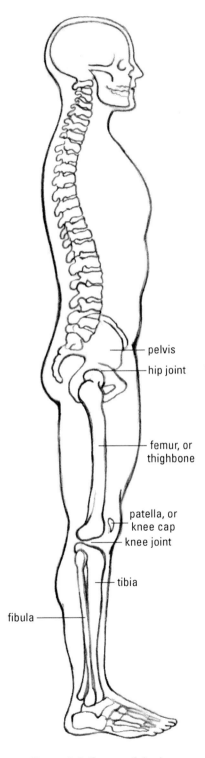

pelvis

hip joint

femur, or
thighbone

patella, or
knee cap

knee joint

tibia

fibula

Figure 3-2. Bones of the leg.

In the saddle, the leg hangs from the hip joint in slight external rotation. This leg position accommodates the horse's barrel. The degree of external rotation will depend upon the rider's anatomy (a narrow pelvis will lead to more external rotation than a wide pelvis), the shape of the twist of the saddle, and the horse's shape (a horse with a broad back will require the rider's leg to externally rotate more than a horse that is slab-sided). This external rotation at the hip joint places the rider's knee gently against the saddle flap supported by the knee roll and places the lower leg against the horse's rib cage. It is appropriate for the rider's toe to point outward slightly, as opposed to facing straight ahead. Because of the knee joint anatomy, pointing the toe straight ahead will place rotational strain across the knee joint, cause the foot to invert at the ankle, or force too much internal rotation at the hip joint, pulling the rider's knee too tightly against the saddle.

This balanced leg position should allow the ball of the foot to rest on the stirrup iron with a sense that just the weight of the leg sits on the stirrup, as if it is on a shelf. That is, you are neither pulling your foot off the stirrup, nor pushing weight onto the stirrup. The weight of your leg will allow your heel to rest below the level of the front of your foot, without force.

We can now add the "heel" part of the shoulder-hip-heel alignment of good rider position (Figure 3-3). The leg rests under the rider's body, hanging from the balanced torso. The ideal leg position would allow the rider to end up standing upright on the arena surface in balance if the horse were taken out from under her.

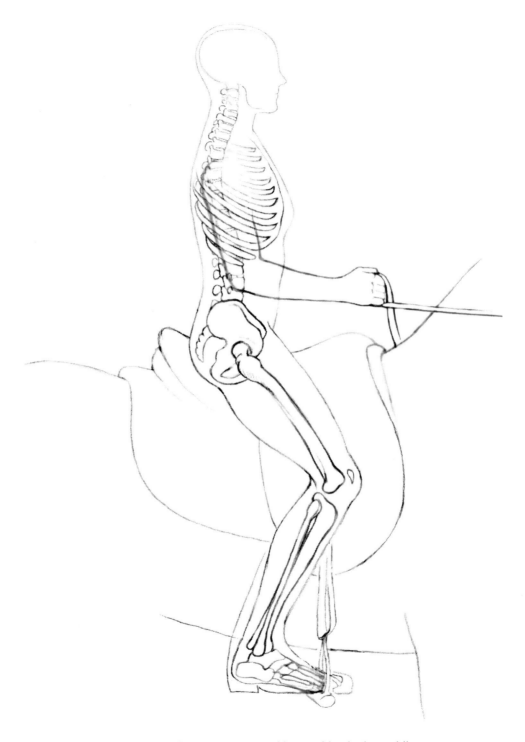

*Figure 3-3. Proper posture and leg position in the saddle
results in alignment of the shoulder, hip, and heel.*

My Challenge: Finding a Horse that Fits

Cautious is a word that best describes my approach to getting back in the saddle after my second surgery for a herniated disk in my low back. I'd been through this before. I'm not sure if I returned to riding too soon after my first surgery or if the second disk herniation was just destined to happen. Nonetheless, I waited about a year after my second surgery to consider riding. And that year was full of conditioning and body training (including, of course, Pilates). Finally I was ready to find out if riding was an option for me.

I started putting feelers out for a potential mount to lease and slowly get back into riding. My criteria were strict: the horse must not have jarring gaits and must not be spooky. It must not be tall so I could avoid lifting and reaching while grooming and tacking up. I needed a reliable horse upon which I could explore strategies to keep my back supported and secure while in the saddle.

A friend told me about a 7-year-old Fjord pony mare, Solana, who needed some miles under saddle to augment her driving career. This sounded interesting. Perhaps this breed could be a good choice for my riding rehab needs.

I met my friend at her barn one sunny afternoon. I was encouraged at how easy it was to tack up this 14.1h pony. We set out on a slow trail ride, and I got a feel for how Solana moved.

After about 30 minutes, my back was getting tight. Solana's back was relatively broad, requiring my thigh to externally rotate at the hip joint. This put my back in a bit of extension, or arch, and caused strain. Solana's short-coupled back put a lot of swing in her rib cage as she walked, causing a great deal of movement in my pelvis and hip joint. The combination of her build and her walk put my body in a less than ideal position to move with her without strain.

So, while her size and temperament were positive features for me, Solana's body type was not.

About nine months later, after having found a more suitable mount to get me back in riding shape, I went horse shopping. Again, I was struck by how some horse shapes did not fit me well. I felt strain in my back whenever I rode a horse with a broad back that put my thighbone in too much external rotation and my spine in extension. A more narrow-bodied horse fit me best. I settled on Bluette, a Danish warmblood mare whose dam was a Thoroughbred. Her relatively narrow conformation fit me well. Her gaits were of good quality and reasonable for me to ride. In fact, several years later, Bluette was my partner at Grand Prix.

If you are looking for a horse and have problems with your back or hip joints, don't discredit the importance of conformation in finding the right mount. Not all horse shapes suit all riders, particularly if you have a physical limitation.

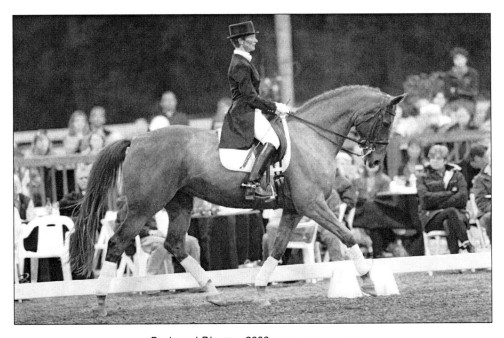

Beth and Bluette, 2006 (Poulsen Photography).

Anatomy of Legs: Hip Joint Muscles

A complex array of muscles connects the leg to the pelvis at the hip joint and operates the knee and ankle joints. Important hip joint muscles are shown in Figures 3-4 and 3-5. Since our legs carry and propel us through the day, our leg muscles are relatively big and strong. Almost as if they have a mind of their own, your legs can demonstrate their excessive strength while you're riding—to the detriment of suppleness and efficiency. Awareness and control of these muscles is vital to allow your legs to move with your horse and give aids of appropriate pressure and timing.

Gluteal Muscles

Figure 3-4 shows the muscles of the back of the thigh. The largest muscle of the body, the gluteus maximus, is one of three muscles that form the gluteal muscles (or "glutes") and the contour of the buttocks. It is a strong muscle, and in conjunction with deeper muscles in the hip, extends and externally rotates the thighbone. When the thighbones are held stable, the gluteus maximus will move the pelvis in a posterior pelvic tilt, or pelvic tuck.

Beneath the glutes is a collection of smaller muscles that rotate the thighbone outward. I refer to these as the deep hip rotators. These muscles help stabilize the rider's leg position in the saddle, working to balance inward rotation and potential gripping from the adductor muscles (see Adductors and Abductors). Many riders benefit from stretching these deep rotators to facilitate freedom in the hip joint.

Hamstrings

The hamstring group of muscles (Figure 3-4) forms the substance of the back of the thigh. This group of three muscles attaches to the seat bone and to the top of the lower leg just below the knee. This muscle group extends the hip joint (it therefore assists the gluteal muscles), and flexes, or bends, the knee.

The hamstrings are a powerful muscle group to access while riding, as they are the muscles that pull your lower leg against your horse's side, as well as pull your entire leg back in the saddle. This provides an efficient and specific tool for your leg aids. The degree to which your lower leg needs to move back to give the leg aid depends a bit upon your horse's sensitivity to the leg aid (which can be trained) and the shape of your horse's rib cage. A sensitive horse will perceive the upper calf against its barrel, requiring little or no lower leg movement when you apply the aid. Others may require a bit more leg contact. It is better to have a brief period when your lower leg is drawn slightly back to give a leg aid than to keep your leg in the same position and pull your calf directly inward. Your knee joint, as a hinge joint, does not allow this inward movement of your lower leg. This can only be accomplished by rotating your whole leg outward. This disrupts the position of both your leg and your pelvis. It is preferable to draw your lower leg back a bit, using the efficient hamstring muscle for a leg aid. Think of directing your heel toward your horse's fetlock of the opposite hind leg. This gives a line of action that activates the hamstrings and prevents your heel from coming up. Your leg must return to its proper position, however, after each aid.

You will access both the gluteal and hamstring muscles in the following pelvic bridge exercises.

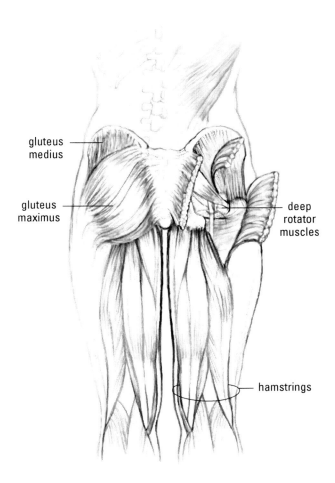

Figure 3-4. Posterior thigh muscles.

Pelvic bridge—simple

All of the pelvic bridge exercises strengthen your hamstrings and gluteal muscles as well as the stabilizing muscles of your trunk.

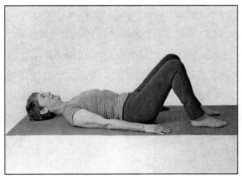 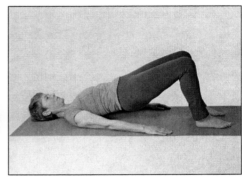

Photo 3-1   Photo 3-2

1. Lie on the floor in neutral spine alignment, knees bent, feet flat on the floor hip joint width apart, arms by your sides (Photo 3-1).

2. Keeping neutral alignment, on an exhale breath, stabilize your spine then activate your gluteal and hamstring muscles to lift your pelvis and torso off the floor, until your body forms a plank from your knees to your shoulders (Photo 3-2).

3. Return your pelvis and torso to the mat, back to start position, as you take an inhale breath.

4. Repeat 6 to 8 times.

I have described doing this exercise in neutral spine, which makes it feel a bit like the motion of posting the trot.

Be sure that the power for this exercise comes from your gluteal and hamstring muscles of the back of your leg. These muscles—not the muscles of your back or arms—lift your body off the floor.

Check that you push off from both feet equally; one leg should not do more work than the other. Keep spine alignment stable and don't let your back arch at the top of the movement; keep your trunk muscles engaged. Don't let your knees fall apart: keep your knees aligned over your feet (placing a small ball or towel between the knees helps).

Pelvic bridge—single leg

This version of pelvic bridge challenges leg strength and the ability of your torso muscles to keep your pelvis level.

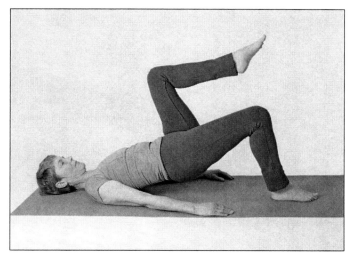

Photo 3-3

1. Lie on the floor in neutral spine alignment, knees bent, feet flat on the floor and close together in the center of your body, arms by your sides.

2. Lift your left knee to your chest.

3. Keeping neutral alignment, on an exhale breath, stabilize your spine then activate your gluteal and hamstring muscles on your right leg to lift your pelvis and torso off the floor, until your body forms a plank from your right knee to your shoulders (Photo 3-3).

4. Return your pelvis and torso to the mat, back to start position, as you take an inhale breath.

5. Repeat 3 to 4 times on your right leg, then repeat lifting with just your left leg.

Try to keep the front of your pelvis level as you lift with just one leg; avoid letting one side dip down. Keep the range of motion small at first. If this exercise causes a hamstring cramp, briefly stretch your leg. Try the exercise again, focusing on improved balance, organization, and smooth movement—this minimizes the chance of a leg cramp.

Pelvic bridge with ball
This version of pelvic bridge adds a balance challenge.

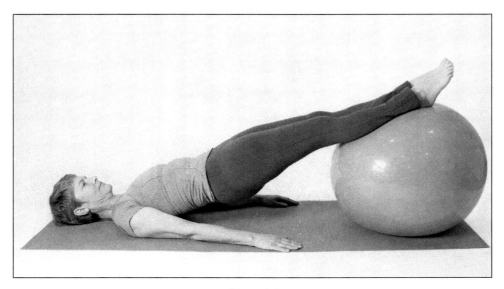

Photo 3-4

1. Lie on your back on a mat with an exercise ball placed underneath your calves.

2. During an organizing exhale breath, stabilize your core and lift your pelvis off the mat so you are a plank from your shoulders to your legs resting on the exercise ball (Photo 3-4).

3. Return to the mat as you breathe in.

4. Repeat the exercise 6 to 8 times.

You will quickly notice the added balance challenge of resting your legs on a ball. Use your core muscles for improved balance. Remember, the ball will roll in the direction of more pressure, indicating you are pressing more on one leg than the other. Try to keep the ball still by lifting equally with both legs. The exercise is easier if the ball is close to your body (thighs or knees on the ball), and more difficult when the ball is farther away from your body (calves or ankles on the ball).

Pelvic bridge with ball—balance

*This version of pelvic bridge adds a balance challenge
by taking away support from your arms.*

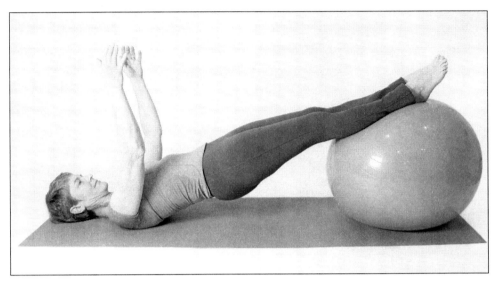

Photo 3-5

1. Lie on your back on a mat with an exercise ball placed underneath your calves.

2. During an organizing exhale breath, stabilize your core and lift your pelvis off the mat so you are a plank from your shoulders to your legs resting on the exercise ball.

3. Maintain normal breathing as you first bend your elbows so your forearms are off the mat.

4. If balance is secure, raise your arms completely off the floor (Photo 3-5).

5. Hold this balanced position for several breaths.

6. Return to the mat.

7. Repeat the exercise 3 to 4 times.

Balancing becomes more challenging when you lift your arms. Work to keep the ball still. Remember, the ball rolls in the direction of increased leg pressure. Use your core muscles for balance, leg muscles for lift.

Pelvic bridge with ball—single leg
Using a ball and lifting one leg adds a balance challenge
to this version of pelvic bridge.

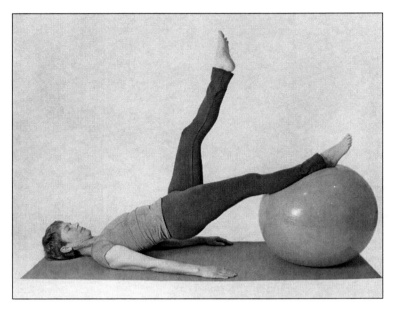

Photo 3-6

1. Lie on your back on a mat with an exercise ball placed underneath your calves.

2. During an organizing exhale breath, stabilize your core and lift your pelvis off the mat so you are a plank from your shoulders to your legs resting on the exercise ball.

3. Carefully shift your right leg toward the center of your body, and either lighten or lift the left leg off the ball (Photo 3-6).

4. Return the left leg to the ball and shift it to the center of your body as you lighten or lift your right leg off the ball.

5. Return your body to the mat.

6. Repeat 3 to 4 times per leg.

Perform this exercise slowly: rushing disrupts balance. Think of "shoring up" the leg that supports you on the ball. Use your core muscles to keep balanced.

Hamstring stretch

This stretch prevents excess tightness of your hamstring muscle, which can affect posture.

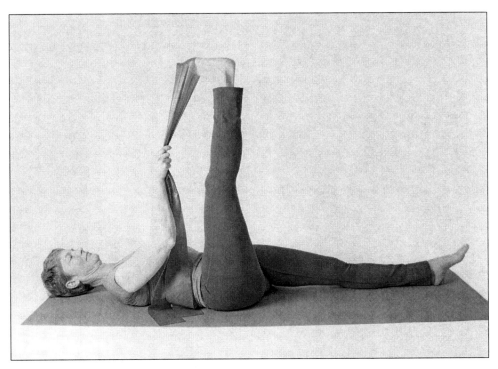

Photo 3-7

1. Lie on your back in neutral spine alignment.

2. Place a towel or elastic band around one foot and reach that foot to the ceiling, working for a straight knee (Photo 3-7).

3. Support your leg weight in the elastic band with your arms, so your leg muscles are not working to keep your leg in the air. Apply gentle traction to your leg—nothing extreme! Do not let your back flatten to the floor.

4. Flex your foot for added calf stretch.

5. Hold for 20 to 30 seconds.

6. Repeat with your other leg.

Hamstring stretch—standing

I prefer to stretch the hamstrings by lying on the floor, as described above. Here is an alternate way to do this stretch, however, if you find yourself in a situation where lying down would be difficult.

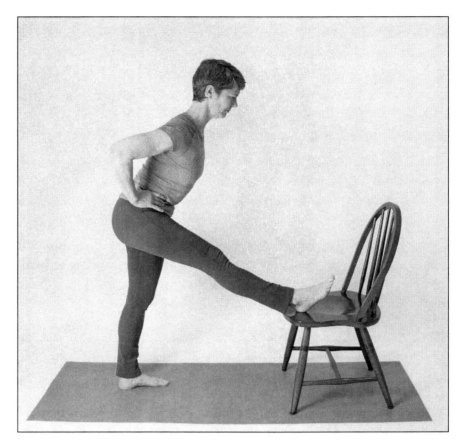

Photo 3-8

1. Standing upright, rest the heel of your right foot on the edge of a chair or an object of similar height. Straighten your leg.

2. Carefully bend your body forward at the hip joint to accomplish the hamstring stretch (Photo 3-8).

3. Hold the stretch for 20 to 30 seconds.

4. Repeat with your left leg.

Do not round your back (Photo 3-9), which avoids the hamstring stretch. Work to keep your back flat or in neutral alignment.

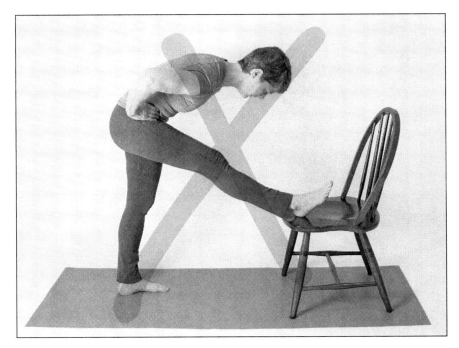

Photo 3-9

Deep rotator, piriformis stretch
This stretch combats tightness in the deep rotator muscles of your hip joint.

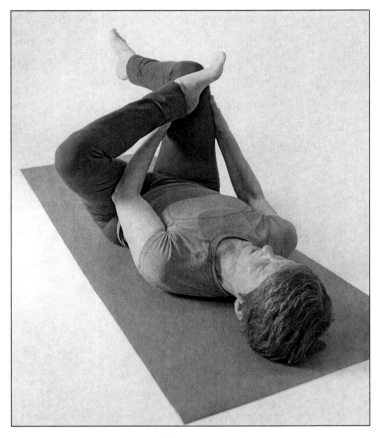

Photo 3-10

1. Lie on your back, knees bent, feet flat on the floor, in neutral spine alignment.

2. Place the side of your left foot on the front of your right thigh, as if crossing your legs.

3. Lift your right leg toward your chest (Photo 3-10). You will feel the stretch deep in the gluteal region of your left leg.

4. Hold for 20 to 30 seconds.

5. Repeat with your right leg.

Deep rotator, piriformis stretch—sitting

This is an alternate way to perform the deep rotator stretch
when lying down is not possible.

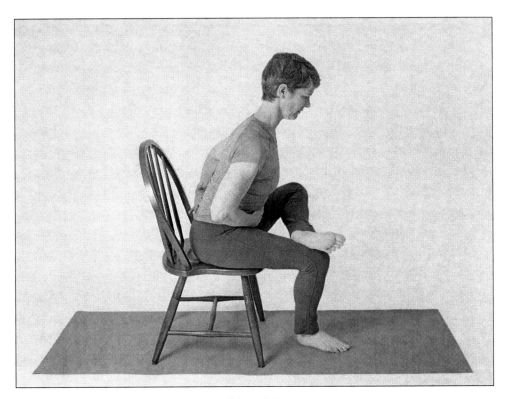

Photo 3-11

1. Sit upright on a chair. Place your left foot on your right thigh, as if crossing your legs. Sometimes this position alone accomplishes a stretch deep in the muscles of your left hip joint.

2. Carefully lean forward from your hip joint (Photo 3-11). This should deepen the stretch in your left hip joint region. Avoid rounding your back as you lean forward; this reduces the stretch.

3. Hold the stretch for 20 to 30 seconds.

4. Repeat with your right leg.

The Rider's Challenge: Overusing Gluteal Muscles
Linda and Wendberg

Linda brings her horse, Wendberg, to the large outdoor arena. The rider's slight build is in distinct contrast to the gelding's stocky frame. During their warm-up, I see Wendberg's blasé attitude force Linda to work and work to keep him going. Linda resorts to using her gluteal muscles to "push" Wendberg into an active walk, with minimal response. Linda pushes harder with her glutes, but Wendberg hardly changes. It is not until Linda gives a thwack with the whip that the gelding becomes lively, at least for a short time. The same pattern appears in the posting trot, with Linda exaggerating the forward thrust of her pelvis at the top of the rise, trying to keep Wendberg moving. And at canter, Linda pushes each stride with a pronounced forward-back movement of her pelvis.

Linda presents a classic picture of a rider working harder than the horse and using her gluteal muscles in a counterproductive manner. Linda understands her dilemma: "I've had such a problem figuring how *not* to use my butt muscles so much. If not them, what do I use?"

I coach Linda to use just her lower leg to get Wendberg going. I suggest a quick, bright leg aid, not a long squeezing one. Wendberg will likely tune out a long squeezing aid, leaving Linda working harder and harder with little to show for her effort. A squeezing aid locks her legs against Wendberg's movement and contributes to his sluggish way of going. I stand by Wendberg's left shoulder facing to his rear and place my hands around Linda's left boot heel. I tell her to give my hands a "leg aid" by using her hamstring muscle to pull her lower leg back. I am careful to not have her do this against Wendberg's side, as she would be giving Wendberg a leg aid without expecting a response from him—and that would be bad training indeed! Linda's initial response is to try and press her lower leg directly into Wendberg's side. This motion causes her leg to externally rotate and her gluteal muscles to fire, and she is pinged out of the saddle. I cue her to think of using the hamstring muscles to pull her leg back, not in. And to minimize use of her gluteal muscles, I have her think of the effort coming farther down on her leg, or closer to the back of the knee. This helps separate the action of the hamstring muscles from the glutes. By imagining her heel being directed toward the fetlock of Wendberg's opposite hind leg, Linda feels her hamstring muscle engage, and I feel a stronger, clearly defined movement against my hands. She is able to give a clear "on" and "off" aid. We repeat the exercise with her right leg.

Back on the rail, Linda practices applying quick and short lower leg aids. This allows her to keep her glutes soft and her entire leg swinging with Wendberg's side. Wendberg quickly learns to respect the quicker leg aid, but when he loses activity and slows down, Linda struggles to not use her glutes. As she practices using her leg in this new way, however, Linda gives a clearer leg aid, lightens her workload, and allows Wendberg to respond with a freer gait.

Exercises for Linda: pelvic rocking supine; pelvic rocking on ball, front to back; pelvic bridge—simple, single leg, and with ball

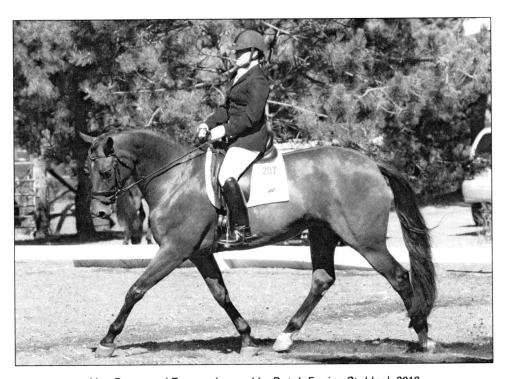

Lisa Boyer and Zamora (owned by Dutch Equine Stables), 2010.

Adductors and Abductors

The adductors and abductors are two muscle groups with opposite action. The *ad*ductors pull the leg to the middle of the body, and the *ab*ductors pull the leg away from the middle of the body.

The adductors are the inner thigh muscles. A group of five strong muscles (Figure 3-5), the adductors attach to the pubic bone and along the inside of the thighbone. The action of the adductors pulls the thigh against the saddle; as such, they are often overused to grip the saddle, like a clothespin. Certainly the adductors are important to stabilize proper leg position, but their role must not expand to include security.

The abductors work in the opposite way: they pull the thigh away from the saddle. As such, they help stabilize the position of the thighbone, or femur.

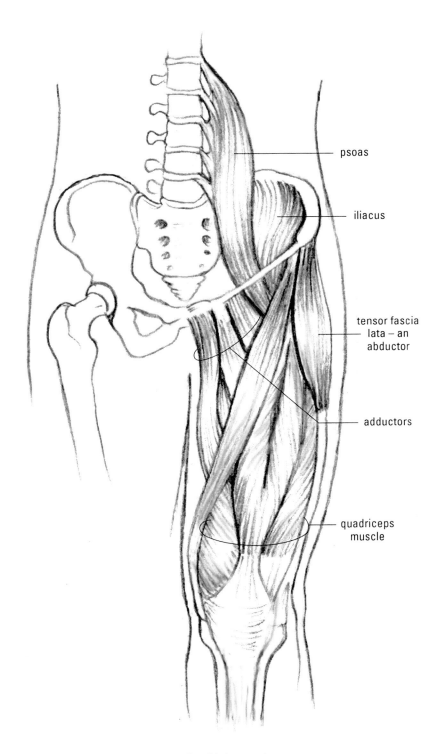

Figure 3-5. Anterior thigh muscles.

Ball tongs—squeezes
This exercise works the adductors (grippers).

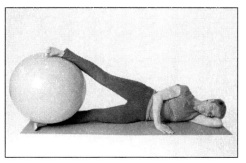 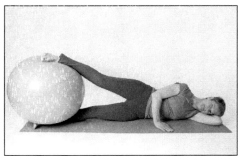

Photo 3-12   Photo 3-13

1. Lie on your left side, holding an exercise ball between your lower legs (Photo 3-12).

2. Rest your head on your left arm on the mat, and place your right hand on the floor in front of your waist for balance.

3. Check that your body is properly aligned, with your shoulders stacked one upon the other and your pelvis lined up perpendicular to the floor. Straighten your legs and place them at a slight angle in front of the rest of your body.

4. On an exhale breath, squeeze the ball between your legs (Photo 3-13), then release the squeeze on the inhale breath.

5. Repeat 6 to 8 times.

6. Repeat lying on your right side.

Be careful that your spine doesn't twist during the leg movements. Keep your weight centered over the left side of your pelvis.

For added difficulty, remove your supporting hand from the mat.

Ball tongs—lifts

This exercise works the abductors (antigrippers).

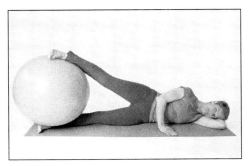

Photo 3-12

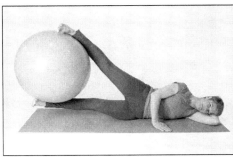

Photo 3-14

1. Lie on your left side, holding an exercise ball between your lower legs (Photo 3-12).

2. Rest your head on your left arm on the mat, and place your right hand on the floor in front of your waist for balance.

3. Check that your body is properly aligned, with your shoulders stacked one upon the other and your pelvis lined up perpendicular to the floor. Straighten your legs and place them at a slight angle in front of the rest of your body.

4. On an exhale breath, lift the ball and legs together off the mat; use your right arm for support, if needed (Photo 3-14). Rest your legs back down on the inhale breath.

5. Repeat 6 to 8 times.

6. Repeat lying on your right side.

Be careful that your spine doesn't twist during the leg movements. Keep your weight centered over the left side of your pelvis.

For added difficulty, remove your supporting hand from the mat.

Adductor stretch

This stretch combats tightness in the adductor muscles of the hip joint.

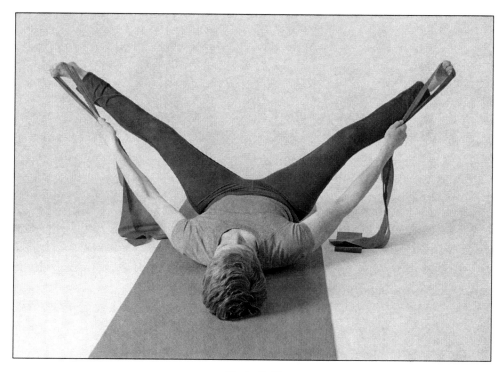

Photo 3-15

1. Lie on your back on a mat.

2. Wrap a towel or stretchy band around the bottom of each foot.

3. Hold tightly onto the towels or bands while reaching your legs together up toward the ceiling, as straight as possible, and then carefully supporting them in a stretch out to the side (Photo 3-15). Be sure to avoid changing your pelvic position during this stretch.

4. Hold for 20 to 30 seconds.

Abductor stretch

This stretch combats tightness in the abductor muscles of the outer hip joint. I often do this stretch right after the hamstring stretch.

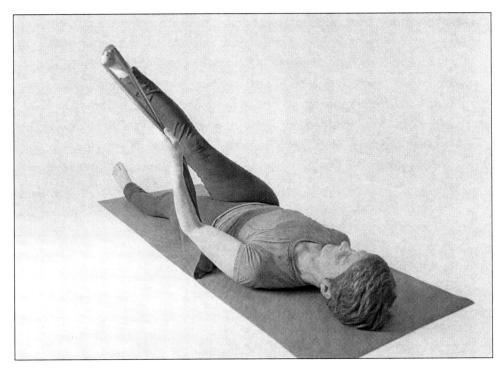

Photo 3-16

1. Support your right leg in either a stretchy band or a towel, holding it with your left hand.

2. Reach your leg as straight as possible to the ceiling (like the hamstring stretch).

3. Let your right leg go left across your left thigh, without much change in your pelvic position (Photo 3-16).

4. Hold the stretch for 20 to 30 seconds.

5. Repeat with your left leg.

The Rider's Challenge: Gripping Adductors
Elise and Peony

Before working with new riders, I ask them to provide some information about their riding experience, goals, and how I might help them. On her form, Elise states, "I don't understand why I get so tired after only riding about 30 minutes. I do not think I'm that out of shape!"

I meet Elise on her 6-year-old bay Trakehner mare, Peony, and watch her do some warm-up rounds at posting trot and canter. She has reasonably correct posture and rides with a very positive "come with me" attitude. However, while the mare will initially pick up the canter fairly readily, before long Peony loses impulsion and breaks out of canter.

"It is so much work to keep her going!" Elise exclaims as she comes back to a walk.

I have Elise do some trot work first to sort out the challenge she has keeping Peony moving in canter. At posting trot, Elise maintains good balance and alignment and stays with Peony. At sitting trot, however, it is a challenge for Elise to keep Peony in a rhythmic and ground-covering trot. I see that Elise's leg gets quite still, too still, and that her back loses its stable position. Her leg position gets so locked that her feet bounce up and down in the stirrup, rather than rest on the stirrup with movement through the ankle joints.

Elise grips hard to keep from bouncing at sitting trot. By doing so, she inhibits Peony's movement, interfering with her staying in a good trot. I'm suspicious that this is also what is going on in the canter. I explain to Elise that her legs should be against the horse, but not gripping. When the legs grip, it is like riding with the brakes on. Peony responds with a loss of steadiness in the trot and a tendency to break out of the canter.

At the halt, I have Elise actively stabilize her spine with her deep abdominal and back muscles, and then carefully lift her legs slightly away from the saddle, out to the side. She immediately feels how much heavier she sits in the saddle, in a good way. I have her repeat the exercise at walk to help her learn the sensation of a more supple, less-gripping leg, and a heavier and more anchored position of her pelvis. I emphasize that it is easy to strain her back with this exercise of lifting the legs off the saddle; it must be done carefully with suitable spine support, aiming for a small range of upper thigh motion, as if she were trying to slide a piece of paper between her leg and the saddle.

Back at sitting trot, I again coach Elise to activate her core muscles and then try a few steps of sitting trot, keeping her legs far enough "away" from the saddle to prevent gripping. She does this for a few steps, and then her legs fire. But she begins to feel when the gripping creeps in.

We do the same exercise at canter to try and get her legs to let go and allow Peony to canter freely. To prevent her legs from clinging to Peony's side, I coach her to give a fairly loose leg aid, being conscious of its beginning and end: apply the aid and then *let go*. I also coach Elise to, at times, give a light tap with the whip, rather than use a leg aid, to encourage Peony to stay in canter. In this way Elise feels her legs stay released and free.

Our lesson lasts about 45 minutes, with a lot of transitions and attempts to keep Elise's leg muscles supple and not gripping at all gaits. At the end Elise remarks, "I don't remember the last time I rode for 45 minutes straight through without a break."

Exercises for Elise: Knee circles, leg circles, leg lifts on ball, adductor stretch

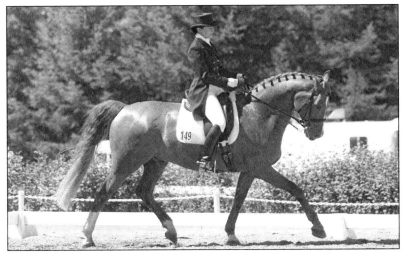

Catherine Reid and Sedona (owned by Sally Kohloff), 2010.

Quadriceps

In Figure 3-5, note the large quadriceps muscle that forms the bulk of the front of the thigh. One of the strongest muscles in the body, this muscle has four parts (hence the name). Its primary action is to straighten the knee, but one part of the muscle crosses the hip joint and can flex this joint (along with the psoas). The quadriceps muscle can interfere with hip joint mobility by pulling the knee up against the knee roll of the saddle. And the quadriceps muscle can disrupt leg position (see "The Rider's Challenge: Unstable Leg Position in Posting" in Chapter 5). The quadriceps muscle does not do much while you are riding. It is not common to straighten the knee joint in the saddle. Two exceptions are the up phase of posting trot, and correcting the position of a lower leg that is too far back.

Straight legs
This exercise strengthens the quadriceps muscle.

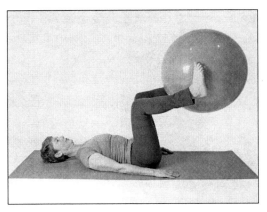
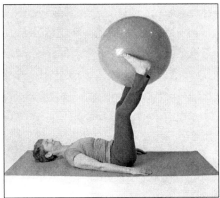

Photo 3-17   Photo 3-18

1. Lie on your back, holding an exercise ball between your feet.

2. Bend your hip joint so that your femur, or thighbone, is perpendicular to the floor, and bend your knee joint so that your lower leg is parallel to the floor. Keep your spine in neutral alignment. Place your arms by your sides or use your hands to support your thighbone position (Photo 3-17).

3. Take an inhale breath, and on the exhale breath, straighten your legs at the knee joint; keep your hip joint stable (Photo 3-18).

4. Return to start position on an inhale breath.

5. Repeat 6 to 8 times.

If your hamstrings are tight, you may not be able to completely straighten your knee joint. This is OK. Do not compensate for this by letting your knees fall away from your body. Be sure to keep your femur perpendicular to the floor so you do not strain your back. Your spine alignment should not change during the exercise.

Psoas Muscle

Figure 3-6 shows the psoas (pronounced 'sō-az) and iliopsoas muscles (for simplicity, I'll call the muscle the psoas). It is a unique muscle in that it is the only muscle that connects the thighbone, or femur, directly to the vertebrae, or spine, at the center of the body. All other thigh muscles connect the femur to the pelvis. The psoas muscle fibers originate on either side of the low thoracic and upper lumbar spine. From there the psoas courses through the pelvis, being joined by the iliacus muscle, to be called the iliopsoas. It then inserts on the femur, or thighbone. The psoas muscle flexes the hip joint (decreasing the forward hip angle) and/or moves the vertebrae of the spine.

The psoas lies deep within the body: it is not easily felt and cannot be seen. As such it is a hard muscle to understand. Those who have tight and restricting psoas muscles have perhaps had massage or physical therapy to loosen the muscle and will know the intense feeling of the muscle being massaged through the abdominal wall.

As a strong and central muscle, the psoas can work for you or against you. When supple and controlled, the psoas muscle offers both spine and hip joint stability with refined control of motion and leg position. This positive function requires control of spine alignment with the postural muscles (discussed in Chapter 2). The knee folds exercise integrates spine stability with psoas muscle function.

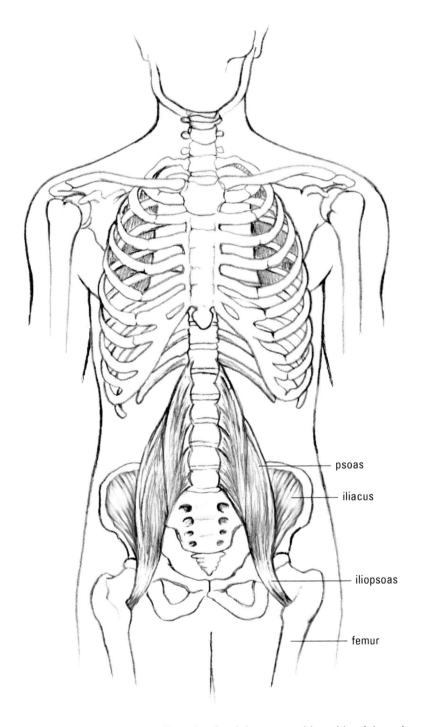

Figure 3-6. The psoas muscle. Note that it originates on either side of the spine, enters the pelvis where it is joined by the iliacus muscle of the pelvis to become the iliopsoas muscle, then attaches to the top of the femur.

Knee folds

*This exercise coordinates the function of the
psoas muscle with your core muscles.*

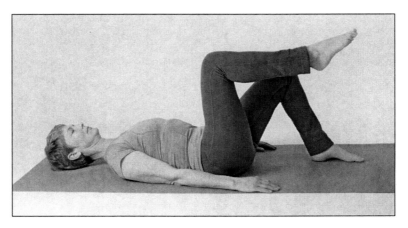

Photo 3-19

1. Lie on the floor, knees bent, feet flat on the floor hip joint width apart.

2. Take an inhale breath, and then exhale and pull in your lower abdominal muscles to stabilize your spine.

3. Lift your right knee toward your chest (Photo 3-19), and set your leg back down without letting your pelvis rock side to side.

4. Do 6 to 8 lifts.

5. Repeat with your left leg.

Engage your trunk muscles to prevent your pelvis from rocking and your weight from shifting while you lift your leg. Pay careful attention to your pelvic position during the exercise, and work for complete pelvic stability with no wiggles.

To access the iliopsoas muscle to lift your leg, imagine that the movement comes from deep within your body's center. Because this muscle is deep within your body and you can't really feel it, you only know you are using it correctly if other muscles work less. You can tell when you access the iliopsoas if the tendon of a more superficial muscle (the rectus femoris) at the front of your hip joint barely tightens during this movement. Check for this by placing your thumbs over the front of your hip joint. When this tendon barely pops up, you are accessing the iliopsoas muscle to move your leg. Also, using the iliopsoas muscle for this exercise confers a stable feeling to your body; it becomes easier to keep the pelvis stable without rocking side to side during the leg lift, and your leg feels like it weighs less.

This exercise is made more challenging by lifting one knee, and then alternating leg positions, so you always have one leg resting on the mat and one leg in the air.

Hip flexor stretch
This stretch combats tightness in the muscles that flex your hip joint.

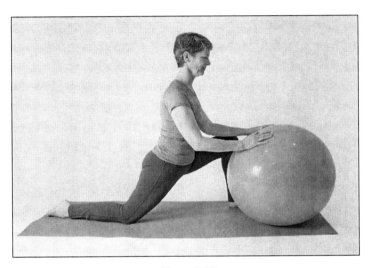

Photo 3-20

1. Kneel on a mat and place your left foot in front of you. You will be resting on your right knee and your left foot. You can use an exercise ball to balance and support your upper body.

2. Press your weight forward over your left foot (position your left foot so you avoid bending your knee more than 90 degrees). You will feel a stretch in the front of your right thigh (Photo 3-20).

3. Hold the stretch for 20 to 30 seconds.

4. Repeat on the left side.

Keep neutral spine alignment and avoid arching your back in the stretch.

The Rider's Challenge: Tight Psoas Muscle

Sarah and Trapper

Sarah jogs up on Trapper as I arrive at her outdoor arena. "I have an important issue to discuss today," she says. "It is embarrassing, but lately after I ride I am sore where I sit in the saddle, and oh my, it hurts to pee after riding!"

Sarah is an advanced beginning amateur rider who recently started leasing this 12-year-old Hanoverian schoolmaster. She is having some difficulty adjusting to his large gaits and learning to stay with his movement.

I watch Sarah at walk and posting trot. Her focus and postural alignment and balance are quite satisfactory. When she tries to sit Trapper's large trot, however, I see her knees pull up and in against the knee roll of the saddle, and her torso comes forward with an arch in her spine. She bounces madly, making the gripping worse. Trapper stiffens his back and loses impulsion.

I explain a little bit about the psoas. I believe her psoas is pulling her thighbone up and pulling her spine forward in an attempt to stabilize her balance. It is not an uncommon strategy, but, unfortunately, it doesn't work well: it pulls her pelvic floor uncomfortably onto the front of the saddle, causes fatigue, and interferes with Trapper's way of going.

I guide Sarah into a more balanced position with her abdominal muscles supporting neutral spine and pelvic alignment. Like a seat belt, these muscles support the pelvis as if it were laced to the back of the saddle. These same muscles keep the pelvis and pubic bone more supported in the front of Sarah's body, preventing the front of her pelvic floor from pressing uncomfortably on the twist of the saddle. As well, I have her seek a more extended hip angle, with her knees staying down in the saddle. With her abdominals pressing back toward her spine and her knees reaching down, she is lengthening the psoas muscle and telling the abdominal muscles to take over the work of balance and support that the overworked psoas has been providing.

Sarah goes back to the rail to try out these changes. She is able to keep her pelvis anchored with her seat-belt abdominals for a few steps, but then she finds herself pitched forward and gripping. It can take some doing to change a habit. I encourage her to try to keep her improved posture for a few steps of a slow sitting trot and then come to walk when she feels herself start to grip again. With practice, she will eventually sit more and more steps, and then a bigger and bigger trot.

Exercises for Sarah: Pelvic rocking supine; pelvic rocking on ball, front to back; knee folds; hip flexor stretch

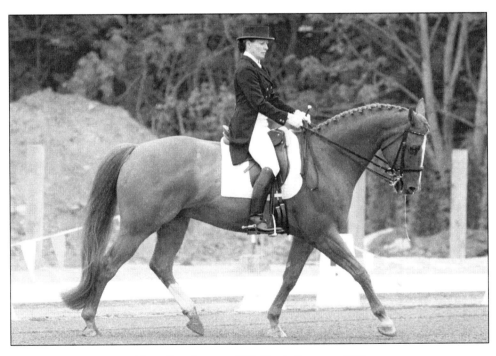

Mary Houghton and W. King's Ransom, 2010.

Leg Position and Function Challenges

In all of us, the weight of the leg comprises a significant portion of our body weight. As such, the legs can have significant unwanted effects on body position and function. Us-

Using the leg to aid the horse can alter posture, and overzealous leg muscles can inhibit the horse's motion.

ing the leg to aid the horse can alter posture, and overzealous leg muscles can inhibit the horse's motion. Finally, leg position can influence our ability to balance efficiently. These are reasons to keep the legs under control and balanced in strength and flexibility.

Leg Dysfunction Affects Posture

Legs can affect posture in several ways.

Applying a leg aid can cause your pelvis to tuck under your body, bringing your spine into flexion or a rounded posture. This is especially true if you tend to overuse your gluteal muscles. This can strain your back because force is being applied with your spine out of neutral alignment. Body awareness and core stability will improve your ability to give a leg aid without such a change in posture. This is one component of independent aids. Work to become aware that leg movement at your hip joint need not change your spine alignment. Off-horse practice will help you differentiate movement of your leg at the hip joint from movement of your pelvis and spine. The knee and leg circle exercises will help you develop this awareness.

A tight and restricting psoas muscle can disrupt position. A short psoas muscle will tend to pull the lumbar spine forward and into extension, or an arch, and pull the hip joint into flexion, narrowing the hip angle (see the example of Sarah and Trapper in "The Rider's Challenge: Tight Psoas Muscle" in this chapter). The rider tends to be pitched forward with seat bones pointing too far back. The antidote for this position problem is finding correct spine alignment, supporting this position with the deep abdominal muscles, and allowing the psoas to stretch and lengthen—to take the work of balance away from the psoas muscle. Then, the knee can move downward, increasing the hip joint angle. The image of kneeling can help you get this feeling in the saddle. The hip flexor stretch exercise in this chapter can teach you this movement off the horse.

If your balance is unsteady, moving your leg to apply an aid can disrupt your position and make it difficult for your horse to understand your cue.

Trunk muscle support prevents this problem. Pay attention to your torso stability while applying leg aids. This may be particularly important when using a strong leg aid. Think of using the opposite torso to counterbalance the leg aid. The leg lifts on ball exercise in this chapter will help you develop this skill.

The Rider's Challenge: Leg Aids Disrupt Posture
Julie and Bismark (continued from Chapter 2)

Remember Julie and Bismark, the gelding that needs motivation to move freely? The first story focuses on Julie's spine alignment, bringing her into a more upright posture with less flexion, or rounding, of her spine. This helps her stay balanced with Bismark's large and lanky trot and prevents her from falling behind his movement. The second issue that challenges Julie's posture is the way she applies leg aids. With each leg aid, her flexed posture returns, complicating her balance.

Julie tends to give a "go" aid to Bismark by squeezing her lower leg against his side, and at the same time, squeezing her gluteal muscles. The gluteal muscles pull her pelvis into a tucked position, with her seat bones pointing forward and her back rounding into flexion. At halt, I remind Julie of correct posture then show her how to apply her lower leg aid just from the hamstring muscle, without the effort generalizing up into her gluteal muscles. In this way she avoids rounding her spine into a potentially harmful position.

"But I always hear 'drive him more from your seat,'" she says. "So what should I be doing?"

I explain that pumping with the gluteal muscles is not the best way to get a sluggish horse moving. I coach Julie to give quick lower leg aids, keeping her gluteal muscles less involved, and to have a clear start and finish to each leg aid so her legs can release. This decreases her work and the likelihood that her posture will be disrupted.

Back on the rail, Julie practices her new, quick lower leg aids. Bismark does not always respond, and Julie then reverts to involving her gluteal muscles and rounding her back. I urge her to use her whip, as opposed to her gluteal muscles, to get Bismark going. Not only will there be clearer consequences to him, but also she'll avoid straining her back by pulling it forcefully out of good alignment.

Exercises for Julie: pelvic rocking supine, knee folds, knee circles, leg circles, leg lifts on ball

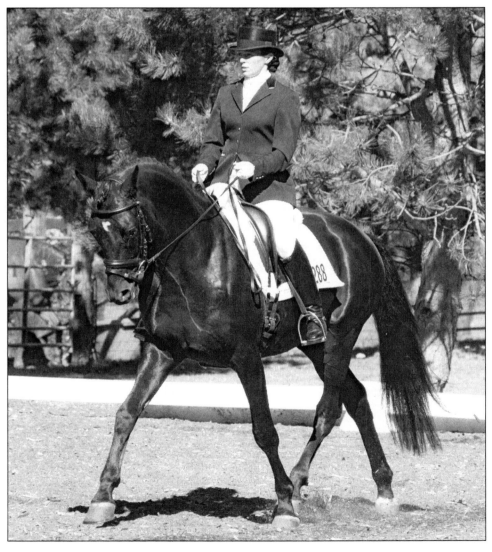

Catherine Reid and Eisenherz (owned by Kathie Vigoroux and Sherry Tourino), 2010.

Leg Dysfunction Is Inefficient

The glutes are hip-joint muscles commonly overused in riding. You can see when a rider is overusing her glutes: she is the one working hard to get her horse to move. Overusing your glutes causes a pumping motion: you tuck your pelvis under as you try to keep the horse going. This problem is most obvious in walk and canter but is also evident in both sitting and posting trots. This pumping is an ineffective method of giving the horse a "go" aid and is sometimes adopted when you are told to "drive with the seat." Using your gluteal muscles to encourage your horse is best reserved for a well-trained and sensitive horse that will respond to a small pelvic tuck. Otherwise you end up working harder and harder, using more and more muscle tone, with little response from your horse and not much to show for your effort. I've seen sensitive horses lock their backs against their rider's tight gluteal muscles with resulting top line tension and loss of purity of rhythm, particularly in the walk. Using your glutes too much also pings you out of the saddle and prevents you from feeling your horse's body move underneath you.

It is overly simple to say that you shouldn't use your gluteal muscles while in the saddle. That is not the case. These muscles assist in leg extension at the hip joint, thus pulling your leg against your horse's side. The point is to avoid using *only* your glutes to get a sluggish horse going. You'll work too hard with little effect. Instead, use a "go" aid from your lower leg and back it up with a tap of your whip; clearly release the aid so your muscles let go, your hip joint unlocks, and your horse can move.

Constantly nagging your horse with leg aids is also inefficient. A lazy horse can coax you into giving a "go" aid with your lower leg every stride. This is a problem of training, one that takes a great deal of rider discipline to correct. Work to have a system of increasing leg aids. Each time you give an aid, start with the little aid, and then increase the forcefulness of the aid until you get a response, perhaps resorting to a tap with a whip. Then, stop giving the aid and expect your horse to continue in the manner that you want. If your horse loses energy, repeat this routine. Breaking the habit of nagging aids requires you to focus on what you want and be consistent in your system of aids.

Sometimes it is difficult to be aware that you are, in fact, giving a leg aid every stride or two to keep your horse going. If you think this is the case, try this exercise for a few strides: Pull your legs very slightly away from your horse's side (to be sure you are not giving aids), and only use a tap with a whip to keep your horse going. This exercise will improve awareness of your leg function, but I do not suggest riding like this all the time, of course. It allows you to feel what it is like for your legs to be supple and released, moving with your horse, and not constantly giving an aid. Try to return to this released feeling each time you use your legs to aid your horse.

How often do you hear "don't grip"? Why is gripping a bad thing? Your leg muscles are strong and can be quite effective, in the short term, at keeping you in the saddle: if your horse bucks or bolts, gripping can prevent a fall. But, otherwise, gripping restricts movement at your hip joint and locks your body against the movement of your horse. This has two undesired consequences: it results in unhealthy mechanics in your body and inhibits your horse's movement.

If you grip, you lock or limit motion at your hip joint, and it cannot move with your horse. Your horse's movement must be transferred into your body someplace, and the likely place is your spine. Gripping can cause excessive and unhealthy movement of your spine. Recall the description of the cushioning disks that lie between each vertebrae of your spine. These disks allow for some movement between the vertebrae, but if your back moves too much, you risk wear and tear on these disks and the intervertebral joints. This is particularly noticeable in the sitting trot. These

By achieving balance and stability in your torso, you support these joints and allow motion to occur at your hip and other leg joints—joints meant to move!

joints can suffer strain and inflammation from the concussion of your body weight if you bounce against the saddle with a locked hip joint. Most assuredly there is some movement at these intervertebral joints while riding all gaits, but if all motion from your horse is absorbed at these joints, you risk strain. By achieving balance and stability in your torso, you support these joints and allow motion to occur at your hip and other leg joints—joints meant to move!

Gripping with your legs for balance works against riding efficiently. While riding, the primary function of your legs is to move with and aid your horse. Your legs should feel part of your horse's body (Figure 3-1). A tight leg makes it difficult to feel your horse's movement, and if your leg muscles are tied up keeping you secure in the saddle, they are not available for small or subtle leg aids. Your horse will experience a lot of "noise" coming from your gripping legs and will be hard pressed to "hear" your leg aids. You, therefore, will need to give an overly strong aid that your horse can perceive over the white noise of your gripping legs. Further, your horse's natural movement involves its body and rib cage. If your legs grip against this movement, you are telling your horse to stop. Essentially, you are riding with the brakes on and, again, this will require you to give leg aids that are perhaps stronger than necessary.

A sure sign of too much leg tone and gripping is fatigue (as in Elise's case; see "The Rider's Challenge: Gripping Adductors" in this chapter). The large leg muscles use a lot of energy. Your leg muscles tire when you use them for both balance and loud, strong leg aids. Transferring the work of balance back to your torso allows you to maintain a secure position, ride with less fatigue, and not work your legs so hard.

Besides causing fatigue, overactive leg muscles impair your ability to sit deeply in the saddle. Have you ever been coached to "sit deep" and wondered how to do this? You cannot push yourself into the saddle, you can sit only as heavily or deeply in the saddle as your body weight allows. However, you have many ways to pop yourself out of the saddle. Tight gluteal muscles push you out of the saddle, and gripping adductor muscles ping you out of the saddle. So when you are told to "sit deep," remind your core muscles to secure balance and take work away from your tight leg muscles. Then, let those muscles release—welcome to your saddle!

Poor Leg Position Disrupts Balance

Your leg position impacts your balance. Proper leg position forms the classic shoulder-hip-heel line. Ideally, your leg is positioned under your body in such a way that if your horse were gone, you would land standing upright on the arena floor.

While you are sitting in the saddle, if your leg comes too far in front of your body, which can happen when you use your feet rather than your pelvis as a base of support, you are placed behind the horse's movement (Figure 3-7). This position is sometimes called a chair seat. If this happens at posting trot, you tend to fall heavily in the saddle in the *down* phase and struggle to keep balance in the *up* phase. Depending upon the degree of imbalance, you may then rely upon the reins for stability. As such, your horse gets a "slow down" or "stop" message from you (often followed by a kick, creating quite an unsteady trot and a very confused horse). This "water ski" position can also happen in down transitions if you push into your stir-rups to support your balance. This body position invites your horse to fall onto its forehand against the bridle. By keeping your leg underneath your body, you are better able to stay in upright balance over your horse's motion regardless of gait or transition. In this position you can act as a conductor for your horse, proactively influencing its movement rather than reacting to what happens after the fact. And, when you improve your balance, you improve your horse's balance.

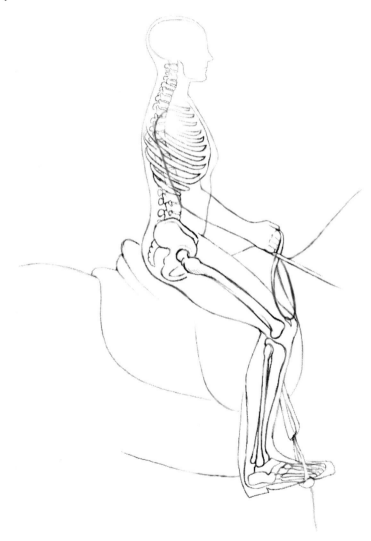

Figure 3-7. This rider is in a chair-seat position. The legs are too far forward, placing the rider behind the motion of the horse. The rider's spine is often rounded, or flexed, with this leg position.

An unsteady leg position that falls behind you also compromises balance (Figure 3-8). If your leg is too far back, your body will pitch forward and you'll find yourself in a very precarious position indeed—one that challenges your ability to keep control of your horse and strips you of your balance tools. In this position, any unexpected movement from your horse can completely unseat you.

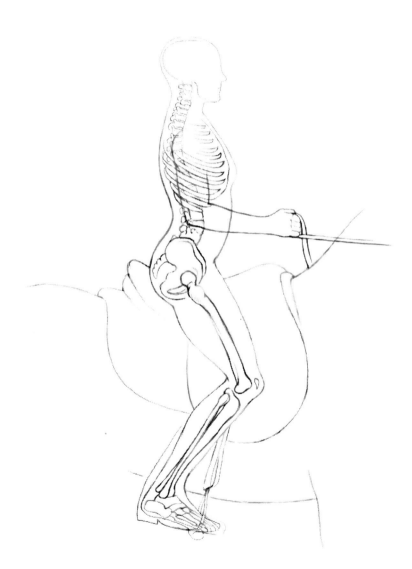

Figure 3-8. This rider is in a perched position, with too much weight on the front of the pelvic floor. The legs are too far back, pitching the rider forward in an unstable and precarious position. This position is often accompanied by an arched, or extended, spine position.

Knee circles

This exercise teaches you to separate movement at the hip joint from movement at the spine, and it improves spine stability and suppleness in the hip joint muscles.

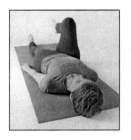 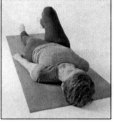 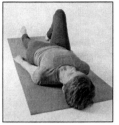 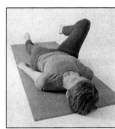

| *Photo 3-21* | *Photo 3-22* | *Photo 3-23* | *Photo 3-24* |

1. Lie on the floor, knees bent, feet flat on the floor hip joint width apart.

2. On an exhale breath and while keeping neutral spine, lift your right knee toward your chest (Photo 3-21). Place your hand on top of your right knee. Straighten your left leg so it is flat on the mat.

3. On another exhale breath, move your right knee in a circle to the left, bringing the right knee over your left thigh (Photo 3-22), away from you (Photo 3-23), out to the right (Photo 3-24), then inhale as you return your knee to the start position.

4. Do 6 circles left, then 6 circles right.

5. Repeat with your left knee.

Use your trunk muscles to keep the pelvis stable, unaffected by your leg movement. Do not allow your pelvis or torso to rock side to side as your leg moves. Gradually let go of your knee and do the circles without the help of your hand (as shown in the photo series).

Leg circles

Leg circles are harder than knee circles and further challenge you to differentiate movement at the hip joint from movement at the spine. Leg circles also improve spine stability and suppleness in the hip joint muscles.

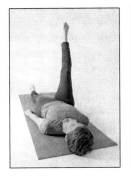 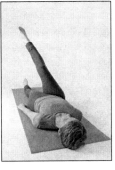 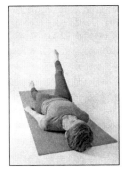 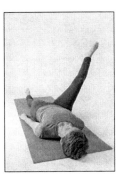

Photo 3-25　　　　*Photo 3-26*　　　　*Photo 3-27*　　　　*Photo 3-28*

1. Lie on the floor, knees bent, feet flat on the floor hip joint width apart.

2. On an exhale breath and while keeping neutral spine, lift your right knee toward your chest. Straighten your right leg as much as possible while keeping neutral spine alignment. Straighten your left leg flat on the mat (Photo 3-25).

3. On the next exhale breath, move the right leg in a circle left, going across the left thigh (Photo 3-26), down toward the floor (Photo 3-27), and slightly out to the right side (Photo 3-28). Inhale as you return your leg to the start position.

4. Do 6 circles in each direction.

5. Repeat with your left leg.

Use your trunk muscles to keep your pelvis stable, unaffected by your leg movement. Do not allow your pelvis or torso to rock side to side as your leg moves. Place your hands on the sides of your pelvis to feel if your pelvis is rocking during the circles. You'll find it particularly challenging to maintain pelvic stability as your leg stretches out to the side.

The knee and leg circle exercises allow you to feel what it is like to have a stable torso and a mobile hip joint with suppleness in these strong leg muscles. Adjust your circle size and keep your pelvis stable while you move your leg. Focus on feeling the stability of your pelvis with coordinated movement of your leg, as you should when riding.

My Challenge: Separate Leg Movement from Spine Movement

It was a huge revelation when, during my Pilates training, I discovered how I had been muddying the movement of my hip joints with the movement of my spine. I had been linking them in a single glob: when I moved or used my legs to walk, lift, or aid my horse, I had no idea that at the same time I was rounding, or flexing, my lumbar spine. I can't say that this caused my back troubles, but I am sure this habitual movement didn't help. It took time for me to learn to differentiate hip joint movement from movement at my lumbar spine. The clear teaching of several patient Pilates instructors helped me sort this out. With this awareness I became better at keeping my spine stable while letting my legs do their job.

Leg lifts on ball

With this exercise you will develop the skill of staying balanced while sitting upright and moving one leg.

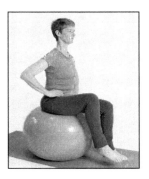

Photo 3-29

1. Sit on an exercise ball or a chair in neutral spine alignment, feet flat on the floor, hip joint width apart.

2. Take an easy inhale breath.

3. On the exhale breath, support your torso and lift your right leg off the floor, with your knee bent (Photo 3-29), then set it back down as you inhale.

4. Repeat with your left leg, then alternately lift each leg 5 times.

Work to keep your body and pelvis stable on the ball or chair as you lift one leg. It requires tremendous torso stability to remain still while you lift one leg. Feel the cross-body balance that happens: as you lift your left leg, feel the muscles of your right torso activate to stabilize the body, and vice versa with your right leg. It is quite normal for your body's coordination to be very different on one side versus the other. Often, lifting the leg opposite your strong side is easier (if you are stronger on your right side, it will likely be easier to stabilize balance when lifting your left leg). If you find it hard to lift one leg without sliding off the ball, think of lifting the opposite pelvis a bit, as you do in the pelvic side-rocking exercise, before lifting the challenging leg. This will activate the opposite torso for stability.

This exercise helps you develop the skill of stability while giving leg aids in the saddle.

The Rider's Challenge: Leg Aids Disrupt Balance
Mary and Bentley

"I'm having trouble getting Bentley into the canter," Mary explains at our lesson. "He just runs off in the trot and I can't stay with him."

Mary is thrilled to have a horse with some training. A 7-year-old warmblood, Bentley is well started and trained to 2nd level. Mary, an intermediate rider, is relearning timing and balance in the saddle after taking a break from riding to start a family. What she lacks in body control she makes up for in focus and determination.

Mary and Bentley move off in posting trot. Bentley gets a bit strong and quick in the trot, and Mary responds by pressing into her feet and "water skiing" against the bridle to slow him down. Her body, as a result, is behind his motion, encouraging him onto his forehand.

I coach Mary to breathe and center and feel more control and balance come from her torso. By getting her feet underneath her body, her balance improves. I have her ride some 15-meter circles to help steady Bentley and create a trot where he stays underneath her.

Mary sits Bentley's trot for a few strides and then asks for the canter. As she had predicted, Bentley runs into a faster trot. Mary's aids are unclear. She thrusts her inside leg forward and turns it out almost as if she were giving an aid to his shoulder. This pushes her pelvis to the back of the saddle; she compensates by leaning forward. Mary's outside leg moves quite far back, contributing to her balance challenge. Bentley, off balance, wonders what to do.

I coach Mary to keep her legs more underneath her body when asking for the canter by applying her inside leg by the girth, not in front of it, and her outside leg just behind the girth. I also advise her to not lean so far forward. She should expect Bentley to canter underneath her.

Mary returns to the rail and tries to modify her leg and body position in the canter transition. While Bentley is still a bit reluctant, Mary's balance is less disrupted and she can more easily correct his running trot. After a few tries, Bentley offers a more prompt canter depart.

Exercises for Mary: Quadruped—single and diagonal, knee circles, leg circles, leg lifts on ball

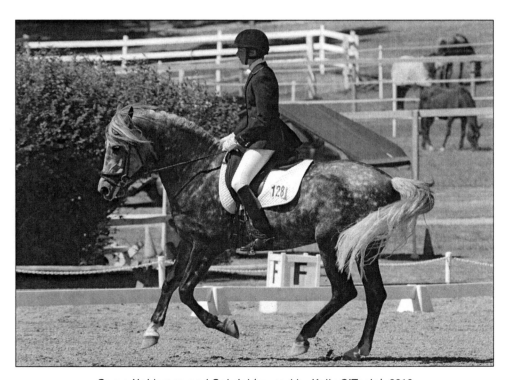

Garyn Heideman and Gabriel (owned by Kelly O'Toole), 2010.

What Is the "Seat"?

You may have noticed that I do not use the term "seat" when talking about rider position issues. I have two reasons for this. First, in my readings I have found variable definitions for the term "seat." I do not want to risk any misunderstanding by using a term that may mean different things to different riders. Second, there are many components to the seat in some definitions:

- *Some use seat to describe your entire position and function.*
- *Some define seat as just your pelvis.*
- *Some define the seat as your pelvis and upper thigh (the body parts you sit on in the saddle).*

The 2011 USDF "Glossary of Judge's Terms" offers this definition of the seat: "The control of the rider's trunk (pelvis, spine, and rib cage, with supporting musculature, not just the buttocks), producing correct dynamic influence, body function, balance, and harmony with the horse's movement (with correct influence/function within each gait and exercise)."

This definition combines some anatomy with function. This definition is quite broad, however, and appears to include the hip joint muscles ("supporting musculature") in the functional unit. I do not like to think of the pelvis and upper thigh as a single unit: I believe that awareness and control of the hip joint, connecting the thighbone to the pelvis, is crucial to good riding.

Also, riders who are directed to "use the seat" often respond by using their gluteal muscles too much. I reserve using movement of the pelvis with the gluteal muscles for advanced and sensitive horses. Before this stage, overusing the gluteal muscles results in the rider working hard with little response from the horse. This issue is demonstrated in these "Rider's Challenge" stories: "Overusing the Gluteal Muscles"/Linda and Wendberg in this chapter, "Leg Aids Disrupt Posture"/Julie and Bismark in this chapter, and "Pumping Gluteal Muscles at Canter"/Sheila and Jade in Chapter 5.

In my experience, the word "intent" can replace some aspects of the term seat. So, when you hear "drive with your seat," you can think of carrying your center of gravity in a forward direction so your body asks your horse for more ground cover, and back up your intent with your leg aids. For many, this is more effective than tucking your pelvis and "pushing" your horse with your gluteal muscles.

Now that you have your legs moving with your horse and more under your control, let's set the same goals for your arms.

CHAPTER 4

Control Your Body: Arms

For most of us, much of our day involves thinking, talking, writing, typing, and generally interacting with the world through our eyes and our computers—running our lives from the shoulders up. This constant use of the eyes and hands can lead to the upper body becoming command central and the arms taking on the role of "control freaks" of the body. Upper body focus leads to the shoulder muscles, rather than the torso muscles, taking over the job of initiating movement and supporting balance. Since they aren't designed for this job, however, shoulder pain, neck pain, and headaches can result.

When on horseback, keeping command central in the upper body and shoulders precludes effective riding. The center of your body, not your upper body, needs to control balance and movement so you can feel what your whole horse is doing. Without this, you risk managing your horse and your ride using information only from what you see, rather than from

The center of your body, not your upper body, needs to control balance and movement so you can feel what your whole horse is doing.

what you feel. And further, you risk making corrections to your horse only with your hands—via the reins—rather than with your whole body.

Relying on your shoulders and arms for balance causes shoulder tightness and a tendency to lean on the reins for stability. Balancing from the reins has obvious and harmful consequences to harmony, as your horse is restricted and feels discomfort from the harsh contact through the bridle. When you correct only with the reins, you risk riding your horse "front to back" and forgetting about the whole horse. Correct rein aids allow, direct, or restrict aspects of your horse's energy and must be delivered with mobility and elasticity, as well as independence between the right and left. Your arms must essentially become part of the bridle, moving with your horse and guiding the energy from your horse (Figure 3-1). This cannot happen if you are using the reins as handles for balance or if your shoulder tension blocks against the movement of your horse.

Anatomy of Arms: Bones

The arms hang off the upper body at the shoulder joint. This joint, like the hip joint, allows a wide range of movements. Via a complex system of muscles, you can move your arms out in front of you, behind you, out to the side, overhead, across your body, and in internal and external rotation. Although few of these actions are desired during riding, keeping the joint mobile and supple avoids rigidity.

Important arm bones include the humerus, or upper arm bone; the scapula, or shoulder blade; the clavicle; the bones of the forearm, the ulna and the radius; and the hand, composed of many bones (Figure 4-1). The elbow connects the forearm to the upper arm. It is basically a hinge joint and is well suited to follow the motion of the horse's neck. The wrist allows many movements, including small refining rein aids. Finally, fingers closed around the reins stabilize rein length.

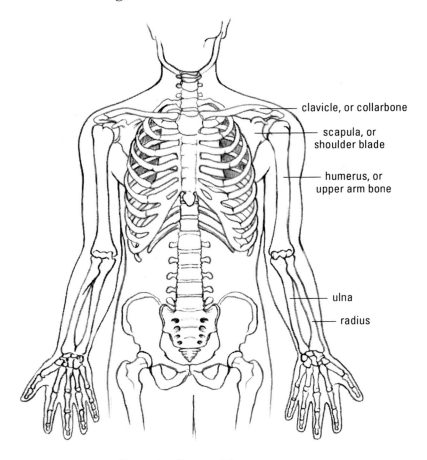

clavicle, or collarbone

scapula, or shoulder blade

humerus, or upper arm bone

ulna

radius

Figure 4-1. Bones of the arm.

Anatomy of Arms: Shoulder Girdle Muscles

The shoulder joint is relatively shallow, compared to the hip joint, so joint stability and alignment depend much more on muscle tone. Figures 4-2 and 4-3 show important shoulder girdle muscles for riding awareness.

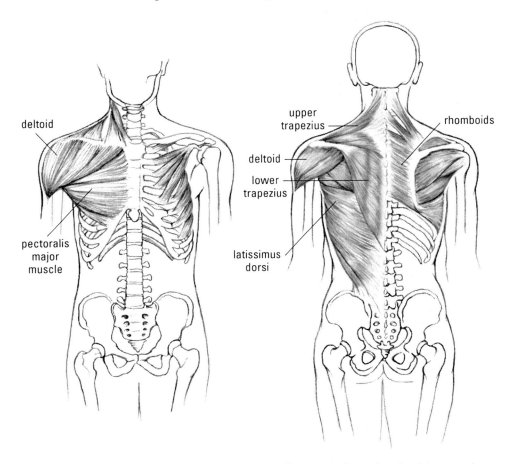

Figure 4-2. Anterior shoulder muscles.   *Figure 4-3. Posterior shoulder muscles.*

The pectoralis major forms the front part of the armpit. This muscle pulls the shoulder forward. Excess pectoralis major muscle tightness rounds the shoulder and can contribute to a rounded, or flexed, posture (Figure 4-4).

Figure 4-3 shows the posterior shoulder girdle muscles. The fan-shaped trapezius can pull the shoulder up into a shrug or back and down in a more desired position. The deltoid forms the upper contour of the shoulder and lifts the arm out to the side.

The latissimus dorsi muscle joins the humerus, or upper arm bone, to the whole of the back, thus connecting the arm to the center of the body. It is one of my favorite muscles for its centering effect. When balanced with appropriate abdominal muscle support to preserve spine alignment, this muscle, along with the lower trapezius, gives the rider great upper body stability. It connects the arm and shoulder girdle to the center of the body, allowing a secure anchor for supple movement. From this comes an elastic connection that doesn't pull, even if the horse tends to be strong in the bridle.

The rhomboids, another important, although smaller, pair of muscles, lie between the medial edge of the scapula and the spine. These muscles assist in pulling the shoulder blades together, and along with the lower trapezius, counteract the unwanted rounding action of the pectoralis major muscle in the front of the shoulder.

Ideally, your arms hang by your sides with your elbows roughly at your waist. Not all riders have the same arm length, however, so elbow position might vary. I encourage a rein length that allows some elbow bend and gives a sense of your hands being out in front of you. Too long of a rein brings your hands back to your abdominal area and restricts their movement. Too short of a rein may result in either pulling or restricting your horse through the bridle, a locked and straight elbow, or a forward position of your torso.

I encourage a rein length that allows some elbow bend and gives a sense of your hands being out in front of you.

Pilates arm exercises improve function of the entire shoulder girdle, making it strong and balanced in its work. Arm exercises teach smooth movement at the shoulder, without disrupting postural alignment. The result is motion that is efficient and appears fluid and easy, like a ballerina's, but, in fact, it requires rider awareness. Exercises develop a strong connection of the arm and shoulder girdle to the torso, allowing the arm to get support and stability from the entire body, and enabling suppleness and elasticity rather than stiffness and grabbing.

Hug-a-tree—both arms

This exercise teaches that your arms can move around your rib cage without disrupting posture, position, or balance.

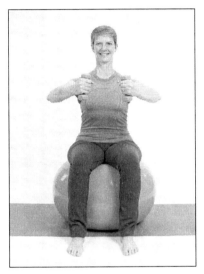

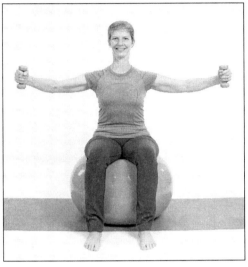

Photo 4-1   *Photo 4-2*

1. Sit upright on an exercise ball, feet flat on the floor, hip joint width apart.

2. Use free weights (the weight should be challenging but not a struggle—I use 2-pound weights in my classes). Raise your arms in front of you just below shoulder height, with your elbows slightly bent, as if "hugging a tree" (Photo 4-1).

3. Take an easy inhale breath, and on the exhale breath, open your arms out to the side (Photo 4-2). Bring them back in front of you as you inhale.

4. Repeat 6 to 8 times.

Keep your elbows lifted, but avoid shrugging your shoulders. Keep the bend in your elbow stable throughout the movement. Do not let your arm movement alter your posture. You might feel a tendency to lean back as your arms come in front of you, and to arch your spine and lean forward as your arms go out to the side. Feel your shoulder blades slide together as your arms open out to the side. This might create a beneficial stretch in the pectoralis muscle in the front of your shoulder.

Hug-a-tree—single arm
This exercise improves balance when you move one arm at a time.

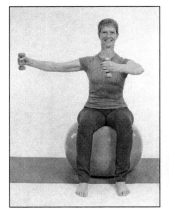 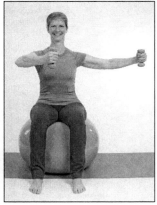 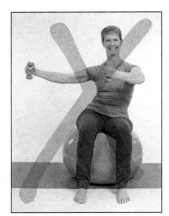

Photo 4-3   *Photo 4-4*   *Photo 4-5*

1. Sit upright on an exercise ball, feet flat on the floor, hip joint width apart.

2. Use free weights (the weight should be challenging but not a struggle—I use 2-pound weights in my classes). Raise your arms in front of you just below shoulder height, with your elbows slightly bent, as if "hugging a tree" (Photo 4-1).

3. Take an easy inhale breath, and on the exhale breath, stabilize the left side of your body while you reach your right arm out to the side (Photo 4-3). Bring your right arm back in front of you as you inhale.

4. On the next exhale breath, stabilize the right side of your body while you reach your left arm out to the side (Photo 4-4). Bring your left arm back in front of you as you inhale.

5. Repeat 3 to 4 times for each arm.

Try to stay upright and steady. You may feel your body try to counterbalance the single arm movement by falling to the opposite side (Photo 4-5). Anchoring the opposite side first helps prevent this and develops the skill of staying balanced when using a single rein.

Chest expansion

This exercise develops a correct shoulders-back position with a stable and supported shoulder girdle, not an arched spine.

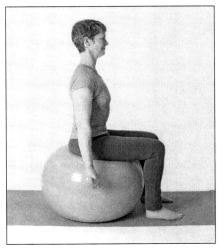 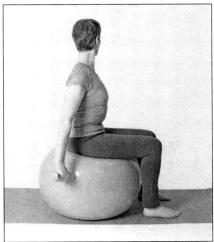

Photo 4-6   *Photo 4-7*

1. Sit upright on an exercise ball or a chair, feet flat on the floor, hip joint width apart.

2. Hold a 2-pound free weight in each hand; let your arms hang down by your sides, palms facing behind you (Photo 4-6).

3. Take an easy inhale breath, and on the exhale breath, reach your arms back by pulling your shoulder blades together.

4. Keep your arms back, and while breathing normally, turn your head to the right and then to the left (Photo 4-7).

5. Return your head and arms to the start position.

6. Repeat 4 to 6 times.

Avoid shrugging your shoulders or pushing your chest out during this exercise. Keep abdominal muscle support so your posture stays stable.

The next two partner exercises illustrate arm skills. I do *not* advise that you always ride in either of the extreme manners illustrated in these exercises. They are meant to define a spectrum of arm mobility and stability. I *do* believe that you need these skills for harmonious and balanced riding. These exercises are described using exercise balls; you can also do them standing.

Partner arm suppleness
The goal of this exercise is to feel how supple and moveable your arms can be.

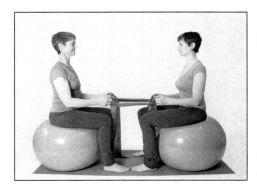

Photo 4-8

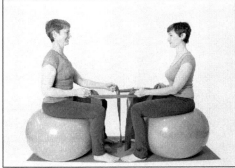

Photo 4-9

You'll need a partner, two exercise balls, and two stretchy bands.

1. Sit on an exercise ball facing your partner, who also sits on an exercise ball.

2. Grasp the ends of the stretchy bands as if holding reins (Photo 4-8).

3. Alternate roles: first, one of you is "horse" and the other is "rider." Have enough contact between the two of you to create slight tension in the stretchy band "reins."

4. If you are horse, move your arms back and forth, not necessarily rhythmically; some randomness is good.

5. If you are rider, keep steady contact with your horse partner by moving your arms while she moves her arms (Photo 4-9). The effect should be even pressure in your "reins" throughout.

6. After a few moments, reverse roles.

Keep the movements slow so steadiness is possible. Feel how you can nearly predict how your horse partner will move her arms, using your focus and balance. Avoid shrugging your shoulders; keep correct posture. Feel the potential for mobility and elasticity in your arms.

Partner arm stability

*This exercise requires body position stability to prevent
a pulling horse from unseating you.*

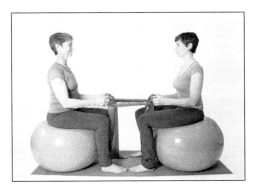
Photo 4-8

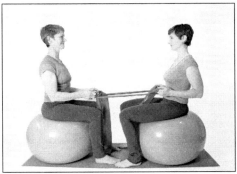
Photo 4-10

For this exercise you'll need a partner, two exercise balls, and two stretchy bands.

1. Sit on an exercise ball facing your partner, who also sits on an exercise ball.

2. Grasp the ends of the stretchy bands as if holding reins (Photo 4-8).

3. Alternate roles: first, one of you is "horse" and the other is "rider." Have enough contact between the two of you to create slight tension in the stretchy band "reins."

4. If you are horse (person on the right in Photo 4-10), gradually increase tension in the band so you are pulling against your rider.

5. If you are rider (person on left in Photo 4-10), keep a steady body position despite your horse's pulling.

6. After a few moments, reverse roles.

When you are rider, prepare for the pulling horse by feeling your arms anchor down your back: think of the V-like lower trapezius and latissimus dorsi muscles. Stabilize your balance by engaging your abdominal muscles. As your horse partner pulls, feel how you can exactly mirror the pulling force by engaging the shoulder girdle and core muscles, so that you are not moved or put off balance by your pulling horse partner. Use an exhale breath to anchor and stabilize your body. Avoid actively pulling against your horse partner; just try to match the pulling force. This allows you to soften and "reward" your partner when she stops the pulling. If you actively pull, when your partner releases you will fall backward out of balance, tugging on your partner. If you are horse, don't be too sudden or strong—you want this exercise to be productive, not harsh.

Partner chest expansion
In addition to stretching your shoulders back, this exercise improves your sense of feel for contact.

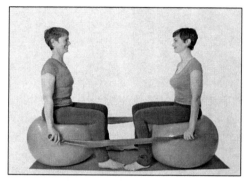
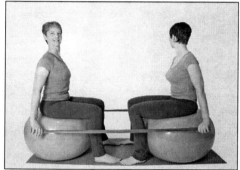

Photo 4-11   *Photo 4-12*

For this exercise you'll need a partner, two exercise balls, and two stretchy bands.

1. Sit on an exercise ball facing your partner, who also sits on an exercise ball.

2. Grasp the ends of the stretchy bands holding your arms straight down by your sides with palms facing behind you (Photo 4-11). Keep enough tension in the stretchy band "reins" so that there is no slack between the two of you.

3. Perform the chest expansion exercise together. Take an easy inhale breath, and on the exhale breath, press both arms behind you and pull your shoulder blades together (Photo 4-12).

4. Hold your arms back and turn your head to the right, and then to the left (Photo 4-12), and then release your arms forward.

5. Repeat 4 to 6 times.

Work to match your partner's effort to keep an even excursion of your arms and your partner's arms. Try to elastically begin and end the movement, tuning into your partner's movement. It helps if one of you calls out the movement, so you can predict when to start.

Avoid pushing your abdomen out in front of you as you press your arms back. Keep your alignment stable and upright.

Shoulder stretch
This stretch combats tightness in the muscles of the shoulder girdle.

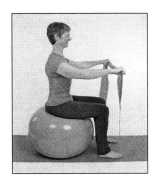 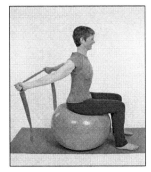

Photo 4-13   *Photo 4-14*

You can do this stretch either sitting on an exercise ball or standing.

1. Grasp an elastic band or a towel with both hands shoulder-width apart, or farther (Photo 4-13).

2. Reach over and behind your head with the band taught to stretch your shoulders back (Photo 4-14). You should feel the stretch in the muscle of the front of your armpit (the pectoralis major muscle).

3. Adjust the stretchy band or towel tension so that you can comfortably lift your arms over your head and behind your back.

4. Repeat the stretch 3 to 4 times.

Avoid pressing your abdomen forward or arching your spine as your arms reach overhead and then behind you. Keep your body balanced.

The pectoralis major muscle is often tight in folks whose lives involve a great deal of desk or computer work. This stretch promotes a correct shoulder position and posture on and off the horse.

Arm Position and Function Challenges

The muscle mass of the shoulder girdle is less than the muscle mass of the hip joint, but it still can influence posture, sometimes in sneaky ways. For example, someone with a computer-based desk job can suffer from a chronically flexed or rounded posture both from sitting all day without proper spine support and from frontward use of the arms causing tight pectoral muscles (Figure 4-4). This postural problem is common. If this describes your work environment, remember to get up now and then to stretch and move and restore good alignment.

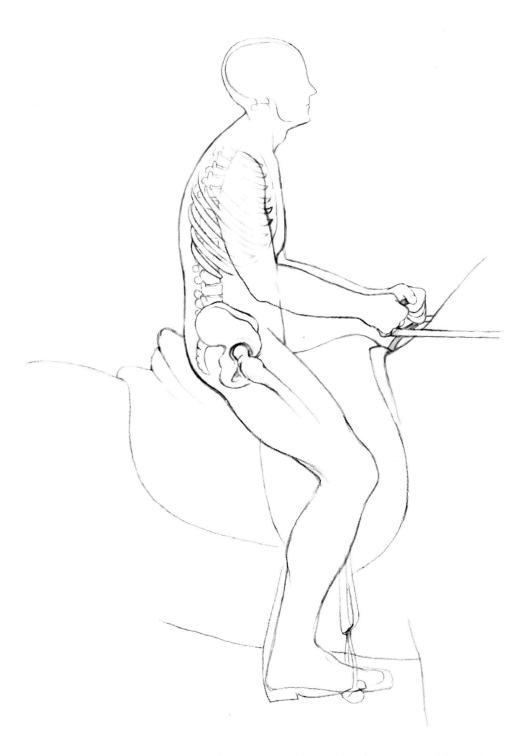

Figure 4-4. The shoulders can disrupt posture. A shoulder that is rounded forward
is very often accompanied by a flexed or rounded posture.

The Rider's Challenge: Rounded Shoulders
Laurie and Mitch

Laurie expresses concern that her lack of stable balance is interfering with the development of her young horse. Laurie is a veteran rider who has explored many disciplines. She recently gravitated to dressage and rides a 5-year-old 16h Dutch warmblood gelding, Mitch. Laurie describes herself as motivated and ambitious, perhaps too much so. And she describes Mitch as mellow.

Laurie warms up at working trot. Mitch's trot lacks activity. Laurie works to keep his trot tempo active by thrusting her body forward at the top of the rise while posting: her gaze drifts downward, her shoulders and upper body round forward, her elbows move away from her sides, and her hands turn in toward her abdomen.

At the halt, I show Laurie a better upper body alignment. However, she struggles to make the appropriate adjustments. When guided to bring her shoulder blades together, stretching her pectoralis muscle, her shoulders lock and her low back arches. This is a common "evasion" in riders with this problem. The shoulders, tight and pulled forward, resist changing position and stretching. From the body's standpoint, it is easier to shift the whole upper body back and arch the lumbar spine than to just move the shoulders around the rib cage. In attempts to correct a rounded posture caused by tight shoulders, the S posture can result.

To help Laurie sort out this issue, I encourage her to think of her shoulders connecting down her back in a V shape (following the latisimus dorsi muscle fiber alignment; see Figure 4-3). At the same time, to avoid an arched spine, I have her feel her rib cage in front remain stable and connected to the pelvis by her abdominal muscles. I describe the upper body and lower body planes used in the S posture correction (see the S-shaped Posture section in Chapter 2).

Laurie struggles with this new position, but determination is on her side. Back at trot, this more upright posture allows her to feel her horse's effort at impulsion, rather than block his energy. There is improved freedom at her hip joint. Her contact through the bridle improves and is more sensitive, as her arms are more supple in this balanced position. She can feel Mitch's energy come from his hind-quarters and flow through her body at the back of her upper thigh, and out in front of her (see Figure 2-1). These subtle but real changes improve Mitch's gait quality and give Laurie a better sense of riding "back to front."

Exercises for Laurie: Spine extension on mat, spine extension—scarecrow, hug-a-tree—both arms, chest expansion, shoulder stretch

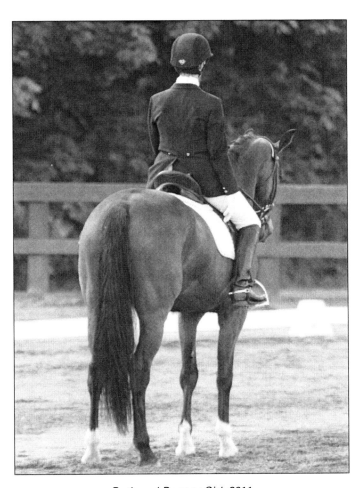

Beth and Donner Girl, 2011.

Riders who carry work and life stresses in their shoulders can end up with a chronic shoulder shrug and extreme tension in the upper body. This muscle tension pulls them up and away from their center of gravity, into an extended, or arched, posture (Figure 4-5). They may experience pain in the mid back because this region is overworking.

Balance and integration of the body for effective riding is difficult with tight shoulders. It is tempting to view tight shoulders as an isolated problem that you can solve by just bringing your shoulders down. Unfortunately, if you follow this cue without a sense of your center, you risk further pulling away from your source of stable balance (your torso), and focusing too much on your arms as the problem (it is most likely your core that is failing).

Remember that what is correct does not feel normal until it becomes a habit.

If this describes you, find your center and allow your shoulders to do less work. But be warned: When you correct this posture, you will probably feel that you are leaning or rounding forward. Remember that what is correct does not feel normal until it becomes a habit. But improving your efficiency of balance and position, as well as gaining support from all the torso muscles (not just those of the mid back), will convince you that the change is a good one.

The improved sense of self and trust in your body gained from improved strength and awareness not only supplies you with concrete tools for stability in the saddle, but also diminishes fear.

Novice or fearful riders often overwork the shrugging muscles (upper trapezius, among others) as their body tries to find some sense of security in the foreign place of being on horseback. This rider must develop a sense of being anchored to the saddle through the pelvis to release the tight shoulder girdle. This problem of self-confidence in the saddle is one particularly amenable to off-horse work. The improved sense of self and trust in your body gained from improved strength and awareness not only supplies you with concrete tools for stability in the saddle, but also diminishes fear.

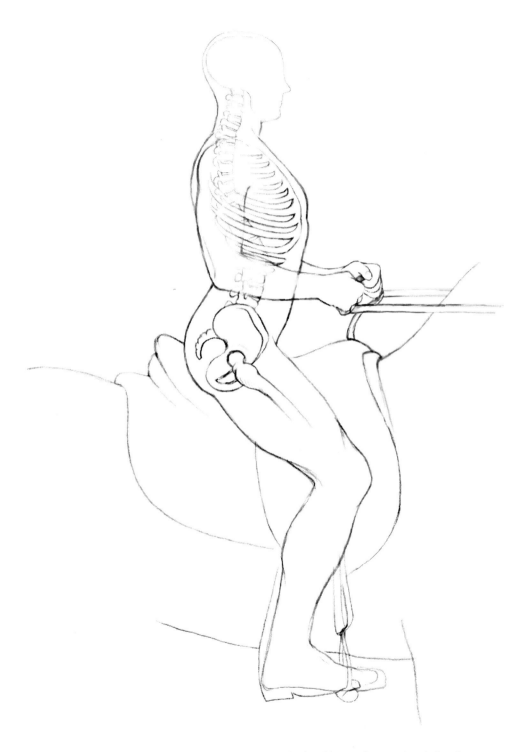

Figure 4-5. The shoulders can disrupt posture. A shoulder and upper back that is tense, with shoulders lifted toward the rider's ears, can cause an arched or extended posture.

The Rider's Challenge: Upper Body Tension
Cassie and Sam

Cassie comes to my Pilates-based small-group exercise classes. She is new to dressage and is thrilled to have a talented warmblood gelding, Sam, who is patient with her learning. She explains that her trainer sent her to my classes to improve her shoulders. "She always nags at me to relax my shoulders. For some reason this is really hard for me to do," Cassie says.

In class, I note that when an exercise requires arm movement, she initiates it by first pulling her shoulders up to her ears. My challenge is to teach Cassie how to move her arms without this obligatory shrug and to help her feel balanced from her torso.

Months later, Cassie comes for a riding lesson. A tall woman with a longish torso, Cassie looks drawn away from her horse with negative tension and energy in her upper body and shoulders. She holds her spine in rigid extension, with seat bones pointing behind her. She draws her legs slightly forward and holds the reins tight as she pilots her horse around the arena by pulling on one rein and then the other, her legs giving a random kick every now and then. She relies on her arms and shoulders to do most of the work.

My goal is to get Cassie feeling the tools of stability within her torso for balance in the saddle. First, we work on breathing to help her get anchored in the saddle and define the pelvis, not the shoulder girdle, as her base of support.

"But I feel like I'm slouching!" Cassie protests as I guide her pelvis slightly back in the saddle to a more neutral position. But when she looks in the mirror she sees how a small change in the position of her pelvis settles her down into the saddle—a very new feeling for her—and contributes to a sense of being connected to her horse's body, not perched on top.

I urge Cassie to focus on her core muscles, feeling a constant hum of connection to these muscles and teaching her brain that they are "there" to support her position and balance in the saddle.

Back on the rail at walk, I coach Cassie to keep the inward stabilizing abdominal muscles in her awareness. When she does this,

I see her release her shoulder tension. She no longer grips the reins like handles, and her contact becomes more elastic and following. Sam responds by lowering his usually inverted neck and reaching to the bit. Confused by the feeling of slouching, Cassie often looks in the mirror to confirm that this changed position is not sloppy. She begins to feel that releasing her shoulders helps her "sit deep," something she had been told to do but didn't know how.

My next client arrives outside the arena, prompting Sam to lift his head suddenly. Cassie responds by reverting to her shoulder-focused control and grabbing the reins. But a centered breath reminds her to release her shoulder tension and sit back down in the saddle.

Exercises for Cassie: Pilates breathing 1 and 2; pelvic rocking supine; pelvic rocking on ball, front to back; abdominal curls; spine stretch forward; leg lifts on ball; shoulder stretch

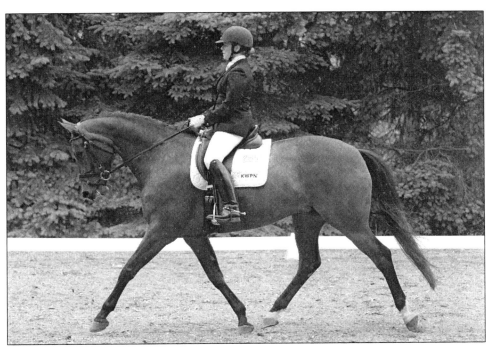

Lisa Boyer and Zamora (owned by Dutch Equine Stables), 2010.

Arms Must Function Independently

Use of your arms for a rein aid must not disrupt your posture, alignment, and balance. This is challenging: in the saddle, your upper body can be relatively mobile, making it easy to lean one way or the other to counterbalance a rein aid. (Think of your body's response to the hug-a-tree—single arm exercise.) But leaning causes an unwanted shift in your weight—confusing your horse. Stability of position starts with balancing from the muscles of your torso. Arm suppleness, mobility, and control are then possible.

The Rider's Challenge: Rein Aid Disrupts Balance
Jeff and Gregor

"I am having so much trouble maintaining bend in the left lead canter," Jeff announces as we start his lesson on his 10-year-old Thoroughbred gelding, Gregor.

I watch Jeff and Gregor warm up at working trot and canter on the right lead. Jeff's posture is fairly good to the right, although he tends to muscle the horse around with his strong legs, rather than follow Gregor's movement. I note that Jeff struggles to control Gregor's right, or outside, shoulder when they trot left. Jeff is "left-sided" and sits to the right as they trot left, overbending Gregor's neck to the inside.

At the left lead canter, Gregor braces against the left rein; Jeff pulls more and falls more to the right. Gregor also falls more and more to his right and eventually stumbles into a hollow, running, unbalanced trot.

Jeff's lateral balance problem is made worse when he uses his left rein. Using his left arm increases tone in his left side and sends him more and more to the right. The more he uses his left rein, the worse his balance gets, until Gregor falls apart. My first goal is to help Jeff feel balanced in the middle of the saddle.

I have Jeff do small pelvic side-rocking movements in the saddle. Not surprisingly, he finds it easy to lift the left side of his pelvis, but challenging to lift the right. While I hold the reins, he practices small spine-twist movements, keeping his seat bones evenly weighted as he turns his upper body. When rotating left, he falls right: I have him lift his right seat bone a bit as he turns left with his shoulders—this helps his balance. While his rightward rotation is initially restricted, it is easier for him to rotate to the right while keeping even weight over his seat bones.

Back on the rail, I have Jeff do some sitting trot figures of eight to help him feel centered going both directions. Rotating his shoulders slightly to the right, or to the outside of the circle, helps Jeff stay "in the middle" when tracking to the left (rather than falling right). While the change feels extreme to him, it is really a simple correction: he stops twisting his body too far to the left. Thinking of turning right keeps his shoulders appropriately aligned with Gregor's shoulders and brings his weight to a more centered position.

At left lead canter, I again coach Jeff to slightly rotate his body to the right. I urge him to avoid using the left rein in such a way that overbends Gregor's neck left, even if this means Gregor is counter-bent for the time being. I also give Jeff my "elbow spur" image for his right elbow (see the Lateral Postural Imbalance section in Chapter 2) and have him turn by bringing his right side to the left. My goal is first for Jeff to feel what it means to not fall right while canter-ing left. When this position feels secure, he can add the bending aids. Until then, however, Jeff's attempts at bending Gregor with his overbearing left rein cause postural problems in Jeff and straightness issues in Gregor.

While it feels awkward for Jeff to engage the right side of his body while going left, the result in Gregor is profound. With his body closer to being straight, he turns left without falling right and maintains the canter on the 20-meter circle.

Exercises for Jeff: Pelvic rocking on ball, side to side; spine twist on ball; leg lifts on ball; hug-a-tree—single arm

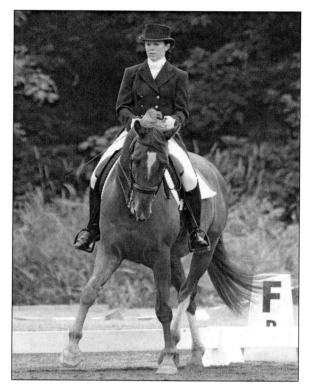

Catherine Reid and Baltic Star, 2010.

Arm Control Facilitates Training

If you need to use more rein as a restraining aid for a strong horse, be careful that your torso position stays solidly upright on the vertical in neutral spine. It is tempting to lean back, press your feet forward, and use body weight to control your horse. This works in the short term and is appropriate for a bolting horse. But to improve your horse's balance, leaning back is the worst thing to do. Leaning back puts you behind the horse's movement and gives the horse something to lean against.

When you lack suitable stability, a strong horse can pull you forward, putting you in a dysfunctional position—perched forward out of the saddle without a base of support—and opening the door to the horse for more evasions. If your horse gets strong, find your base of support by anchoring your pelvis to the saddle with your core muscles and anchoring your upper arms by your sides (think of those latisimus dorsi muscles!). From this position your rein aids are functional and are more likely to make positive changes in your horse. I am not suggesting that you ride around and around with your horse hanging on the reins, but if you let your horse change your position, you have lost effectiveness. Work to keep a stable position when your horse pulls; meanwhile, do exercises and transitions geared toward improving its balance.

Some trainers coach riders to "keep your hands still!" But this cue can be confusing. Your hands *should* move sometimes, depending upon your horse's gait (see Chapter 5). *Steady* is a better word to describe hand position: you control where your hands are at all times. Think of it this way: if you had a pressure meter between the reins and your fingers, the pressure would stay quite stable. Clearly, your horse has some role in this goal! And so do you. Keeping your hands steady develops a quiet connection.

Arm position can reveal balance problems. An arm that persistently "feels" compelled to cross over your horse's neck is likely adapting for a problem with your body's balance and alignment. If you sit heavily to the left when tracking right, you may find the need to cross your left, or outside, hand over your horse's neck to try and control its bulging left shoulder. This arm position is not desirable. Notice what your arm is doing and try to change alignment by improving your balance and position. If you sit heavily to the left while tracking left, you might find your left arm trying to "hold up" your horse's left shoulder by coming up and in, crossing over your horse's neck. Again, note this faulty arm position and realize it reflects a balance issue. Work to sort out your balance so your arms stay in a correct position.

Your hands and arms must not be dead weight on your horse's mouth; rather, you must keep your arms in self-carriage, just like the rest of you. Otherwise, your horse will feel backward pressure on the reins. To keep a sense of your arms being "alive," imagine a current running through a loop defined as follows: from the bit in your horse's mouth, to the right rein, to your hand holding the right rein, to your right wrist, forearm, elbow, and upper arm, then across your upper back and down the left upper arm, elbow, forearm, wrist, hand, left rein, and back to the bit in your horse's mouth. This loop of current must remain unblocked. Unnecessary tension in any part of your arm, such as from a cocked wrist, a locked elbow, or a shoulder shrug, will block current through this loop, and elasticity will be lost.

Do not equate soft and elastic contact with loose fingers on the reins. Loose fingers allow the reins to easily slip out of your hands, causing you to lose steadiness in the contact. Keep your fingers closed on the reins, making your arm part of the bridle. Elasticity and soft contact comes from suppleness in your whole arm, not just in your fingers. Certainly your horse feels an increase in squeeze on the rein: just be sure you do not let go of the squeeze so much that you let go of the reins!

Movement at your elbow is key to maintaining a steady contact with your horse's mouth, especially in the walk and canter, in which your horse's neck undulates as part of the mechanic of the gaits. To keep steady contact, you must allow movement of your elbow joints, as well as your shoulders, so that your hands move with your horse's mouth. At the trot, however, your horse's head and neck are quite steady, while its body (and your body) moves up and down. At this gait, your elbows must allow your body to move up and down while your hands stay steady; your hands should *not* go up and down (see the Trot section in Chapter 5).

A simple example demonstrates the importance of arm muscle suppleness in preserving elastic contact: Hold a cup of liquid in your right hand and walk around. The liquid will not slosh around much because your supple arm adapts for the movement of your walk to keep the cup level. Now tuck something under your right upper arm and walk around. You will see the liquid slosh around madly as your locked upper arm and elbow can no longer move. (I discovered this while carrying the morning paper under my arm with a cup of coffee in my hand.)

Wrist suppleness allows you to fine-tune your connection with your horse when giving aids. With correct arm position and elbows close to your sides, position your hands with thumbs on top, pointing slightly toward each other, with your wrist joint straight. For subtle rein aids, move your wrist by flexing it or bending it inward. Return to start position after each aid.

The Rider's Challenge: Locked Elbows
Jessica and Lambo

Jessica trots over after her warm-up with frustration showing on her face.

"He is always looking away with his head up, totally ignoring me," she says. And to prove her point, this 8-year-old Morgan gelding, Lambo, looks left and whinnies.

Jessica and Lambo walk off. Lambo's walk is tense and quick, with a lateral tendency. He is above the bit, and his well-developed under-neck muscles suggest that this is how he usually moves. Jessica responds to his high-headed posture by pushing her hands down so far that her elbows straighten and her wrists lock. Lambo slows a bit, but his head remains high. A quick kick from Jessica quickens his pace but worsens his tension and walk rhythm.

Jessica is willing to see what happens when she lets go of the reins. Lambo stretches his head out and down, and his walk rhythm improves.

I explain to Jessica that her arm position contributes to Lambo's inverted posture. It may seem like a good idea to put your hands down when your horse puts its head up, but, in fact, it only makes your horse's inverted posture worse!

While I hold the reins with one hand, with my other hand I place Jessica's arm in the correct position for a steady contact with Lambo. I then move her arm forward (toward the bit) and back (away from the bit) but always on a line straight to the bit, showing how her arm should move with Lambo's neck. When she shoves her hands down, it is impossible to have a pleasant connection with Lambo through the bridle. Certainly Lambo has his own issues, but Jessica's job (as the thinking member of the horse-rider team) is to avoid contributing to his issues and then try to sort them out.

Back at the rail at walk, Jessica rides on a longish rein. I coach her to slowly take up contact, little by little. When she gets close to having some contact, Lambo begins to tense. I have her guide Lambo on a circle line and avoid pressing her arm down, but feel it move back and forth with his head and neck movement. He softens a bit to the slight contact. His tempo slows somewhat, but I urge Jessica to not make a big deal about it right now. Our goal is to improve the harmony between horse and rider. I want Jessica to feel how her stiffness is preventing Lambo from moving freely.

We go back and forth from walking on a long rein to gradually taking up contact on a bending line going both directions, with Jessica fighting her habit of pushing her arms and hands down in a locked position whenever Lambo's head comes up. I encourage her to continue staying with Lambo's head and neck movement by moving her arms back and forth. Over time, Lambo becomes less worried about her taking up the reins, and he responds with less tension. Jessica begins to feel how the rhythm of his walk informs the movement of her arms to stay with his head and neck so contact is more sympathetic.

Exercises for Jessica: Pilates breathing 1 and 2, leg lifts on ball, partner arm suppleness, hug-a-tree—both arms and single arm

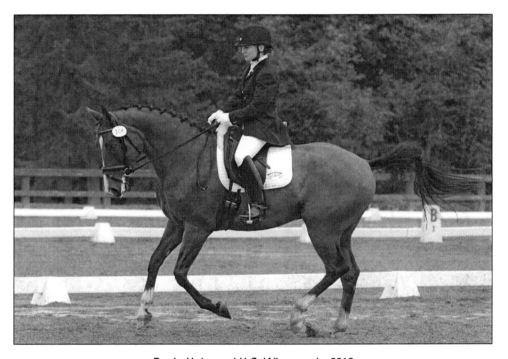

Paula Helm and H.S. Whrapsody, 2010.

With focus, balance from posture and postural support, and control of your "muscle-men" legs and "control-freak" arms, it is now time to consider your horse: next we will explore how you should move with your horse at each gait and transition to promote balance and harmony.

CHAPTER 5

Understand How Your Horse Moves

The final Rider Checklist skill considers the basic characteristics of your horse's gaits and how your body moves with each gait. A simple understanding of your horse's gaits is necessary for you to positively influence your horse's movement. In this chapter, you'll review the three gaits—walk, trot, and canter—and for each gait you will learn "what moves and what shouldn't move much" in your body. Finally, we will cover strategies for improving balance and using your body efficiently and effectively in transitions and lateral movements.

Considering how the horse moves opens the door for riding in harmony: it is the horse's chance to come to the table with its point of view, so to speak.

Considering how the horse moves opens the door for riding in harmony: it is the horse's chance to come to the table with its point of view, so to speak.

For without considering the character of the horse's gaits, we have no basis from which to improve the horse's way of going. The horse's character of movement is its raw material for us to work with. We must understand how we interact with this material before expecting it to change.

The ability to move in harmonious communication with your horse is the same as riding with "feel." Some say feel is a skill you either have or don't have: if you are so lucky to be a rider with feel, you are admired. If, however, you are told you lack this skill, it seems you are doomed to a riding career of struggles.

A rider with feel predicts and interacts with the horse's movements and behaviors as if she can read the horse's mind and body. A rider with feel always appears *with* the horse despite challenges or evasions from the horse. This rider seems to always know just the right amount and timing of encouraging or correcting rein or leg aids, and seems to be sitting inside the horse, rather than on top of the horse. The resulting picture, to the uneducated eye, looks as if the rider is doing nothing (but we know otherwise!).

Young riders have a particular knack for feel. With relatively little guidance, a skilled young rider develops the ability to move with the horse and influence it in a positive way. This is not surprising, as learning new movement skills comes naturally at a young age. As we get older, it becomes harder and harder for the brain and body to learn new tasks and make logical choices for balance and coordination. It is not that we can't learn something new; it just takes longer and requires a greater commitment. If you are an older rider and think you lack feel, don't give up. I strongly believe it can be learned and developed.

The tools provided in this Rider Checklist are what you need to develop feel. First, a proactive mind-set (Chapter 1) allows you to precisely sense your horse's deviations from the desired character of a gait or transition. Balance (Chapter 2) and body control (Chapters 3 and 4) give you the tools to avoid interfering with your horse's movement. Finally, learning and understanding your horse's rhythm and movement at each gait, and how you, the rider, should move with them puts you and your horse on the same page, and the door is open to ride with feel.

Walk

The walk is a four-beat gait. The order of footfall is right hind (RH), right fore (RF), left hind (LH), left fore (LF), as shown in Figure 5-1. There is no moment of suspension at the walk; the horse always has at least two legs on the ground. Therefore, there is no "bounce" or impulsion in the walk, unlike trot and canter.

Walk: What moves and what shouldn't move much

- Your shoulder and elbow joints move to stay with your horse's head and neck.
- Your legs swing slightly in and out at the hip joint, staying with your horse's rib cage as it rocks side to side with each step.
- Your pelvis and spine move somewhat forward and back (but this is often exaggerated). The amount of movement of your pelvis when you ride a walking horse is similar to the amount of movement of your pelvis when you walk.

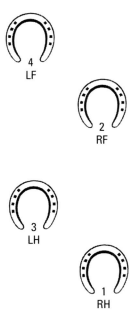

Figure 5-1. Walk footfall diagram (LH = left hind, RH = right hind, LF = left fore, RF = right fore).

The alternate stepping of the horse's hind legs causes its whole body to move. As the horse's RH steps under its body, the rib cage swings to the left. As the horse's LH steps under its body, the rib cage swings out of the way to the right. This causes a side-to-side rocking of the horse's rib cage and back, directly under where the rider sits. Watch a horse walk away from you and you'll see this side-to-side rib cage swing (it is particularly obvious in a fat horse or a pregnant mare). Watch a horse from the side and you'll see the back dip down and up as the hind legs step alternately under the body. While the degree of swing in the rib cage varies depending upon scope of the walk and the horse's conformation, it is there, to a certain degree, in all horses.

Learning the rhythm of the walk and how your horse's body moves helps you sit precisely with your horse. When a hind leg steps under the body, you will feel your thighbone on the same side dip slightly down or in and your opposite thigh lift up slightly. The hip joint on the leg that is lifted up extends open a bit. With practice, you'll feel the alternate hind legs stepping by perceiving the slight rocking of your legs from side to side, and you will start walking with your horse. When exploring this movement, be careful not to create the movement in your body, but let your horse's body move yours. The movement is not huge, but if you do not allow your legs to swing in this way, in essence, you are telling your horse not to walk. You must support the rhythm and character of the walk to be clear to your horse that this is what you want. Every step.

Feel how the rocking of your horse's rib cage moves your thighbone at your hip joint, rather than at your pelvis. Your pelvis most certainly moves slightly during the walk, both side to side as well as front to back and in rotation, but it is easy to exaggerate this pelvic movement and end up moving more than your horse. I encourage some pelvic stability so it stays balanced over your horse's movement.

Now that you feel your legs swinging with your horse's walking steps, you can learn to identify which of your horse's hind legs is stepping under its body. You can check yourself by either looking in a mirror or watching your horse's shoulders (the foreleg on the same side will immediately follow the hind leg). Why learn this skill? Your horse's hind leg can be influenced only when it is off the ground and not bearing weight. It is off the ground when it steps under its body. By knowing when each hind leg steps under your horse's body, you can improve the timing of your leg aids. It is much more likely that your horse will respond appropriately if you ask for more forward reach or a sideways step when its leg is in the air. Stated another way, if you ask for a sideways step from a hind leg when it is on the ground and bearing weight, your horse cannot respond to the aid and will either tune out or resist. Awareness of the stepping hind legs puts precision in the timing of your aids and is a key element of feel.

Awareness of the rhythm and stepping of your horse's legs in the walk also helps you maintain steady activity in the walk. Call out the stepping of your horse's hind legs and keep a steady tempo of these steps marching in your head like a metronome. For simplicity, limit the counting to the hind legs (1-2-1-2) as opposed to all four legs (1-2-3-4-1-2-3-4). With this background rhythm, you will quickly perceive when the horse's energy or tempo changes, and you can give small urging or restraining aids to keep the gait steady. This puts you in a positive and proactive "ride what you want" mind-set while you *appear* to be doing very little. This organization is far preferable to large, obvious, and unbalancing corrective aids.

The horse's neck and head undulate at the walk. Again watch a horse at liberty and you will see how the head and neck move as part of the walk—the horse's mane will swish back and forth. This is the horse's natural gait. You must allow this movement by avoiding stiff and still arms: your arms must move at the elbow and shoulder joints to keep contact through the bridle elastic and steady. Your horse should not be punished each step by hitting the bit. The amount of your horse's movement and, hence, your arms will depend upon your horse and the character of its walk. Test yourself to see if you are suitably staying with the movement of your horse at the walk by trying to maintain an even pressure on your fingers from the reins during all steps of the walk.

When it comes to riding the walk, the most common problem I see is the horse training the rider to work too hard! I see this in two ways: first, the rider overuses the gluteal muscles, and, second, the rider gives driving leg aids every step of the walk. Both are sort of "wishful thinking" walking that makes you work harder than

Your horse's part of the bargain is to walk; your part of the bargain is to expect the walk and stay balanced and rhythmic with your horse, reinforcing the walk you want.

your horse. Your horse's part of the bargain is to walk; your part of the bargain is to expect the walk and stay balanced and rhythmic with your horse, reinforcing the walk you want.

The Rider's Challenge: Working Too Hard at Walk
Susan and Jasper

I arrive at the clinic site and meet Susan, who is warming up her 7-year-old Swedish gelding, Jasper. The horse is clearly unfocused in the new environment, but Susan tactfully goes about helping him settle by riding bending lines and transitions. She is clearly a focused and pleasantly empathetic rider. Her posture and balance are reasonably good, but her aids at times cause tension.

"Sometimes I feel Jasper and I are not on the same page. I try to be tactful, but I feel that my aids often disrupt his way of going and communication is a struggle," Susan explains. "Sometimes he tries to listen, and other times I don't have his attention at all."

My plan for Susan is to review "what moves and what shouldn't move much" at each gait so she can feel more a part of Jasper's body and apply her aids at a logical time. We start at walk.

I watch Jasper initially walk actively on the track. After a few moments, his energy fades and he looks up and hollows his back. Susan squeezes her legs against his sides to urge him forward. He doesn't answer but continues looking away, remaining quite hollow. She adds more leg squeezing and tucks her pelvis a bit as she tries to get him to walk on, tightening her gluteal muscles and pumping with her butt. Jasper remains hollow and further tightens his back against her aids. His walk gets quick, tense, and pace-like, losing its clear four-beat rhythm.

In this circumstance, the timing and nature of Susan's aids are not effective and disrupt Jasper's way of going. Her leg aids are not rhythmic and are applied against his movement. Her tight and pumping gluteal muscles cause further tension in Jasper's back.

I review with Susan the characteristics of the walk. I lead Jasper (so Susan needn't worry about steering or energy) and Susan feels the swing of her legs with Jasper's rib cage. I encourage her toward less back-front movement of her pelvis and more side-to-side swinging of her legs at the hip joint. This helps her pelvis remain quiet and helps her feel the walk rhythm. I then give the reins back to her, and she tries to keep the rhythmic movement in her body.

When Jasper's walk begins to fade, I coach Susan to give smaller, quicker, and more rhythmic aids from her lower leg only, without using her gluteal muscles much. Further, I guide Susan to use her leg to ask for more energy when Jasper's respective hind leg is stepping under his body and is in the air, not when it is bearing weight: that is, her right leg asks for more walk as Jasper's right hind leg swings under his body, and her left leg asks for more walk as Jasper's left hind leg swings under his body. I also have Susan count the stepping of Jasper's hind legs (1-2-1-2) so she mentally and physically walks with him every step.

With Susan's more organized approach to encouraging an active walk, Jasper maintains a rhythmic gait with less tension, and his ears turn backward, listening to her. Susan gives smaller aids to keep an active walk, as she quickly perceives when the walk loses energy. Mentally, she works harder to feel what is happening, but physically she doesn't have to work as hard because her aids are well timed.

Exercises for Susan: Bounce in rhythm 1-4, leg circles, leg lifts on ball

Trot

The trot is a two-beat gait with a moment of suspension between each beat. The horse's legs move in diagonal pairs: RH with LF, and LH with RF, as shown in Figure 5-2. While the walk carries the horse and rider forward, the trot carries the horse and rider up as well as forward—this increased energy at the trot challenges balance in the novice rider.

Trot: What moves and what shouldn't move much

Posting Trot

- Your hands stay in a stable position.
- Your legs stay stable underneath your body.
- Your torso is in stable alignment while it moves up and forward over the pommel of the saddle, and then back down.

Sitting Trot

- Your hands stay in a stable position.
- Your torso is in stable alignment.
- Your hip joints allow the side-to-side swing of your legs with your horse's barrel.
- Your ankle joints move to absorb the up-and-down motion.

Just as in the walk, in the trot the horse's hind legs move alternately. As such, there is the same side-to-side swing of the horse's rib cage and back. This will be discussed in more detail when we consider strategies for sitting the trot (see Sitting Trot in this chapter).

Unlike the walk, at the trot your horse's head and neck carriage is quite stable. As such, your hands need to stay relatively still. That is, if you could put a measuring stick from your hand to your horse's neck or withers, the distance would remain constant during the trot (assuming a reasonably steady head and neck carriage on the part of your horse). Your horse's head and neck lack the back-and-forth movement seen at walk and canter. A common problem in the trot is your arms and hands "posting" up and down or bouncing during the sitting trot. This will antagonize the connection with your horse, and you will be unable to give subtle rein aids. The trot requires you to move your body in the up-and-down motion of the trot while keep-

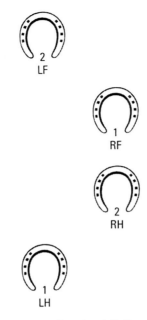

Figure 5-2. Trot footfall diagram.

ing your hands still. This happens when your body is balanced and there is suppleness in your shoulder and elbow joint muscles.

Tuning into the stepping of your horse's hind legs is very important at the trot, as horses are often unsteady in their tempo. Feeling and riding a steady metronome-like 1-2-1-2 rhythm from your balanced center, or core, facilitates a stable tempo in your horse.

Posting Trot

In posting trot, your torso comes forward over the pommel of the saddle and then back down into the saddle in the trot rhythm. It is traditionally taught that you rise out of the saddle when your horse's outside foreleg and inside hind leg are stepping forward and are in the air, and you sit in the saddle when the opposite diagonal pair are stepping forward. The rise out of the saddle is accomplished by extending (angles at the joints increase) both knee and hip joints; then flexing them (angles at the joints decrease) as you return to the saddle. Neutral spine alignment is maintained during the posting trot.

A correct and stable leg position is important during posting trot. With the shoulder-hip-heel line in place in the down phase, the stirrup acts as a platform for you to step onto in the rising phase. Your leg must stay stable under you to provide a support for the rising phase of the posting trot. Without a stable leg position and correct posture, balance is difficult and you risk falling either behind or ahead of your horse—at worst using the reins for balance, and at best ineffectively guiding your horse's trot.

Posting trot has some similarities to the pelvic bridge exercises (presented in Chapter 3). The movement is similar: the focus of the power for the lift comes through the back of the upper thigh, balanced by the torso. However, little power needs to come from you: the horse provides the energy to lift you out of the saddle. But when you precisely direct it through your body, you maintain balance.

A common problem seen at posting trot is an unstable spine position with restricted movement at the hip and knee joints. If hip and knee joint movement is restricted, excessive movement and instability of spine alignment results. When considering "what moves and what shouldn't move much" in the posting trot, the vertebrae of the spine should move very little with respect to each other; the bulk of the movement for posting comes from the hip and knee joints. You know this is happening when the distance between your rib cage and your pelvis stays the same throughout the posting trot cycle. While the spine stays in neutral alignment, there is, at posting trot, a slight forward position of the entire torso. But this forward position comes from a change in the angle at the hip joint, not from a change in spine alignment.

The Rider's Challenge: Unstable Leg Position at Posting Trot
David and Winchester

David asks for help with balance on his new horse. Winchester is a 12-year-old 17.1h Hanoverian gelding that has shown through Prix St. Georges. David has ridden much of his life, mostly casual trail riding. In recent years he has been studying dressage and purchased this schoolmaster to advance his dressage education.

I watch the two of them warm up. Winchester is a big horse with somewhat lanky gaits, but his temperament is very steady. David rides with a positive and fun attitude, although his lack of attention to detail creates a disorganized picture.

We start working on the posting trot. David adopts a common pattern. As he rises out of the saddle, his feet come forward (his knees straighten). This puts his center of gravity behind his horse's motion, and he falls back heavily in the saddle, sometimes hitting Winchester in the mouth. Winchester responds by slowing his trot and bracing his neck. David kicks Winchester on, but his unstable leg position while posting results in his falling back again, and the cycle continues.

At the halt, I hold Winchester's reins and have David rise out of the saddle, as if posting. This is hard to do! Thinking of the pelvic bridge exercise helps David get the power for the lift from the back of his thigh, or hamstring muscles. He first has to hang on to Winchester's mane to rise up out of his stirrups, because he does not keep his feet stable underneath him. When I hold one of his feet in a stable position underneath him, David feels how much easier it is to rise out of the saddle. Gradually I stop supporting his foot and he is able to let go of the mane. To clearly demonstrate what has been happening to him while posting, while David is out of the saddle (still at halt), I move one of his feet forward—and he immediately falls back in the saddle.

Back out on the rail at trot, I have David access the feeling of a stable foot underneath his body as well as the lift of his body out of the saddle coming through the back of his upper thigh in the hamstring muscle region. This allows him to stay in better balance, and his center of gravity stays with Winchester's motion. As a result, contact through the bridle is much steadier, and Winchester can trot forward more freely.

As a final challenge to test his stability at posting trot, I have David rise out of the saddle and stay up for one extra beat (essentially changing his posting diagonal by staying out of the saddle for an extra beat rather than sitting an extra beat). First I have him grab the mane with one hand so any loss of balance is not transmitted to Winchester by pulling on the reins. He finds it remarkably challenging to find the correct balance point at the top of the rise so that he can stay there for a beat. But once he finds it and repeats the exercise without holding onto the mane, his overall balance at posting trot vastly improves, and Winchester's trot settles into a steadier rhythm.

Exercises for David: Pelvic bridge series

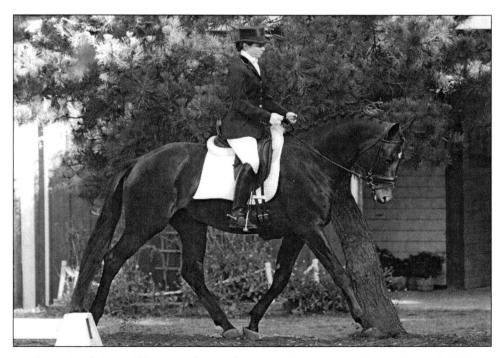

Catherine Reid and Eisenherz (owned by Kathie Vigoroux and Sherry Tourino), 2010.

The Rider's Challenge: Unstable Spine at Posting Trot
Rebecca and Tipper

Rebecca, a high school student who is passionate about dressage, spends every extra moment of her busy life at the barn riding her horse—or anyone else's horse that needs some exercise—and helping out with chores. Occasionally, however, she complains to her mother that her back is sore after riding. Her mother contacts me to see if I have any thoughts about what could be causing the strain. Of note, Rebecca is 5'10" and weighs about 120 pounds. While many admire her long legs, her long torso is a challenge to support.

I watch Rebecca ride the 7-year-old Thoroughbred gelding, Tipper. Rebecca has a positive approach and, in general, a good sense of where her body should be. As I watch her warming up in posting trot, however, I see how her mechanics are not doing her spine any favors.

Rebecca adopts a pattern of posting that accomplishes the back-and-forth movement of her body during posting by moving at the intervertebral joints of her spine, rather than at the hip and knee joints. As a result, her hip angle, which should open in extension at the top of the rise, moves very little. Instead, at the top of the rise, her abdomen presses forward and her spine arches into extension. Her spine rounds, or is flexed, when she returns to sitting in the saddle.

I explain to Rebecca the importance of maintaining spine alignment and moving at hip and knee joints to accomplish the posting trot. As with David (see "The Rider's Challenge: Unstable Leg Position at Posting Trot" in this chapter), I have Rebecca practice the posting trot movement at the halt. It is difficult for her to feel that her spine is doing most of the moving. It is only when I move her pelvis forward over the pommel that she begins to feel that her hip joint can move when she posts out of the saddle. I have Rebecca place her hand on the front of her abdomen to get a sense of the distance between her rib cage and pelvis. She begins to feel that she lets this distance get too long as she posts out of the saddle (arching or extending her spine), and then lets this distance get too short as she returns to sitting in the saddle (rounding or flexing her spine). Keeping her hand "calipers" on her abdomen for feedback, she begins to keep more stability in her spine alignment and find greater freedom of movement in her hip and knee joints.

I guide Rebecca to feel the energy from the horse coming into her body through the back of her upper thigh (hamstring region). Previously, she was feeling and gaining the lift of her body mostly through her low and mid back. This strategy not only is inefficient but also could contribute to her back pain.

Back on the rail, Rebecca practices feeling freedom in her hip angle and a more stable alignment in her spine. All goes well until Tipper gives a little spook, at which point Rebecca's legs grip and she loses the movement at the hip joint. Now, however, she feels the change in her body and goes back to a more supported posture.

Exercises for Rebecca: Pelvic bridge—simple, plank on mat—knees and feet, plank on ball, quadruped—single and diagonal, leg circles

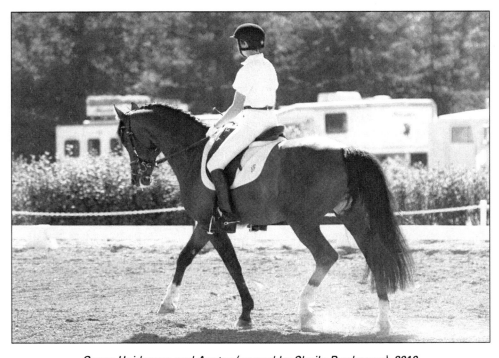

Garyn Heideman and Avatar (owned by Sheila Buchanan), 2010.

Bounce in rhythm 2—arm swings

Bouncing to a metronome is a great warm-up exercise and hones your ability to keep a steady tempo. The added arm and leg movements develop balance and coordination, as well.

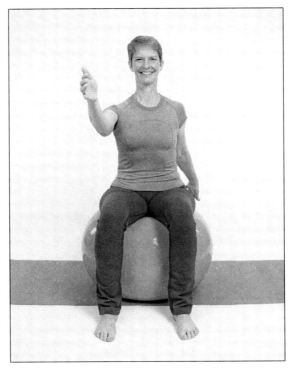

Photo 5-1

1. Set a metronome to about 92 to 98 beats per minute, or put on some music with a similar beat.

2. Sit on an exercise ball in upright posture (as you do for bounce in rhythm 1, in Chapter 1).

3. Bounce to the beat of the metronome or music.

4. Add a rhythmic, alternate, front-and-back swing of your arms (Photo 5-1).

Work for precision: stay absolutely with the beat. Try to land the same way on the ball each time. For variation, try these other movements while bouncing:

Bounce in rhythm 3—toe tapping

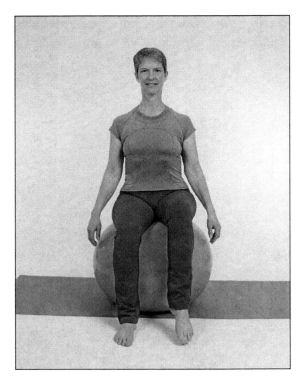

Photo 5-2

1. Continue bouncing to the metronome.

2. Keeping your arms still, lift one leg a bit, and tap the foot in rhythm with the metronome (Photo 5-2).

3. Try to keep your balance on the ball using your core muscles so that moving one leg does not disrupt your alignment (like on the horse!).

4. Once you gain steady balance tapping one foot, change to tapping the other (you'll probably find it easier to tap one foot compared to the other).

5. When this is straightforward, add tapping one foot for a set number of beats, then switch and tap with the other foot.

6. End by alternating foot taps, like marching.

Bounce in rhythm 4—ball jacks

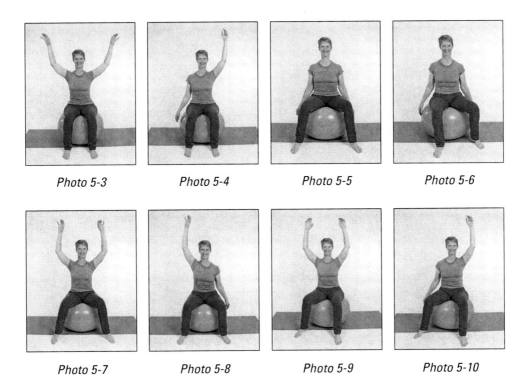

| Photo 5-3 | Photo 5-4 | Photo 5-5 | Photo 5-6 |

| Photo 5-7 | Photo 5-8 | Photo 5-9 | Photo 5-10 |

1. Continue bouncing to the metronome.

2. Swing both arms overhead and back down by your sides, like the arm movements of a jumping jack, for several bounces (Photo 5-3).

3. Next, alternate the swinging of your arms (Photo 5-4).

4. Then, with quiet arms, move your legs out to the side and back in with the metronome rhythm (Photo 5-5). Keep your knees aligned over your feet. Do this several times.

5. When this is stable, alternate your legs: your right leg stays in front of you while your left goes out to the side (Photo 5-6), and vice versa.

6. Finally, combine the arm swings and leg jumps together, like jumping jacks (Photo 5-7). For more challenge, move your arms alternately (Photo 5-8). Then move your legs alternately (Photo 5-9). Then move both arms and legs alternately (Photo 5-10).

With some of these movements, you will probably notice that it seems like the metronome tempo changes. Isn't it interesting how challenging it is to keep a steady tempo, even in the controlled setting of sitting on a ball? These exercises develop coordination, balance, and your ability to maintain a steady rhythm and perceive subtle deviations from what is desired so you can support your horse in steady gaits.

The Rider's Challenge: Use Balance for Tempo Control
Leslie and Sprinx

Leslie asks me for help riding her Morgan mare, Sprinx, in dressage. I explain that my focus is on her more than her horse. "I'm open to any input," she replies.

I watch the two do some trot circles and see that Leslie finds it difficult to keep Sprinx in a steady trot. Sprinx tends to run in the trot, getting quicker and quicker until Leslie pulls on the reins, shoving her feet forward, pushing her pelvis back in the saddle, and then leaning her torso forward out of balance. When Sprinx quickens, Leslie makes dramatic changes in her position such that she is out of balance. This makes Sprinx's trot worse.

At halt I show Leslie a balanced leg position and torso alignment. I teach her Pilates breathing to keep her focused on maintaining balance from her body's center. I explain how she can use her breathing and balance to stabilize Sprinx's trot, with help from the reins, rather than pushing her feet forward. Until Leslie can keep a more stable body position, she will not be able to control Sprinx's trot.

Back on the rail, with Leslie's leg positioned underneath her correctly aligned body, I have the two of them proceed in a slow posting trot. I coach Leslie to count the trot steps and to try to keep her body moving in a stable tempo, unchanged by Sprinx.

Leslie successfully counts the steps for about a half circle, then Sprinx speeds up: she loses focus on the tempo, pushes her feet forward, pushes her pelvis back, leans her torso forward, and pulls on the reins. I point out to Leslie how Sprinx's changing trot changes her.

Leslie is frustrated by Sprinx's behavior, but sticks with it. We go back to counting trot steps while Leslie struggles to break her habit of becoming unbalanced with Sprinx's unsteady trot tempo.

Sprinx snorts her annoyance at Leslie's improved presence. While Sprinx struggles to change Leslie, Leslie remains resolute in her steady rhythm and position. After a few trot circles, Sprinx begins to come around and trot with a much steadier tempo and better balance.

Leslie demonstrates two important factors necessary for good riding. First, do not let your horse change your position, and second, ride the gait you want, not the varied gait your horse offers. Be clear in your own mind about the gait you want, and put yourself in the rhythm and tempo of that gait. Your horse, with practice, will match you.

Exercises for Leslie: Bounce in rhythm 1-4; pelvic rocking on ball, front to back; leg lifts on ball; hug-a-tree—both arms and single arm

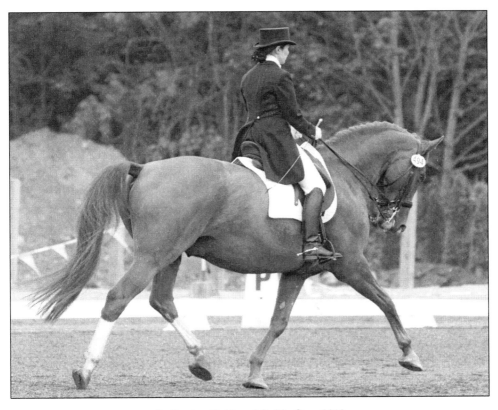

Catherine Reid and Baltic Star, 2010.

Sitting Trot

Sitting the trot is a most challenging skill for a developing rider. It is the gait most likely to trigger detrimental balance strategies, such as gripping with the legs and tightening the shoulders.

I have four strategies to help master sitting the trot:

- **Don't fight the bounce.** Don't try *not* to bounce. Most everything you'll try will make the bouncing worse. Recognize that the trot has up-and-down movement to it. Rather than not bouncing, think of lifting your body up and forward with the horse. And remember, the bouncing you experience rarely looks as bad as it feels.

- **Maintain correct alignment and self-carriage in the trot.** Rather than waiting for the horse to lift or send you out of the saddle, lift yourself up with the horse. Think "trot with me" to the horse, rather than trying to protect yourself from the movement of the trot. Use the metronome in your head to count the 1-2-1-2 stepping of the horse's hind legs to proactively stay with the horse as opposed to being tossed about by the horse. Emphasizing the *up* phase of the sitting trot promotes this self-carriage and sense of trotting with the horse. Focusing on staying *down* in the saddle is rarely a successful strategy.

- **Use the seat belt-like tool of the deep abdominal muscles** to help anchor your pelvis to the back of the saddle so you go up and down with the saddle. Like laces stitching the front of your lower abdomen to the cantle of the saddle, your deep abdominal muscles provide an effective and positive tool to help you stay with your horse at sitting trot. Plus it is something to tell your body to *do*. So often we are saying *don't*: "don't tighten the shoulders," "don't grip with your knees," and so on. But your arms and legs are trying to keep you in the saddle by gripping. Until you replace gripping with an alternate and successful strategy—focusing on your abdominal seat belt—this tension will remain. The abdominal muscle stability organizes the rest of your body so that you can recognize and reduce unnecessary tension. When using this abdominal seat belt, however, avoid changing your spine alignment into a pelvic tuck—stay in neutral spine alignment.

- **Find the side-to-side rhythmic swing of your horse's body to move with it in a positive way.** This swing of your horse's barrel, or rib cage, is similar to what happens at the walk. The challenge, however, is that the sitting-trot tempo is much faster than the walk tempo. It takes practice to feel and stay with this rapid motion. As in the walk, I emphasize the movement of your thighbone at the hip joint with this swinging to help keep a stable pelvic and torso position. Again, it is not that the pelvis is immobile, but it is easy for it and the spine to move too much in the sitting trot.

As you develop the sitting trot, focus on the first three techniques: when core stability, balance, and rider self-carriage are secure, then the hip joint swinging generally follows. Feeling this movement at the hip joints is another positive place for your energy and focus—it is another "do this" strategy. You will not be able to feel your horse's back swing at sitting trot if your legs are tight and gripping.

In my experience, because of the quick trot tempo, it is much easier to explore your horse's swinging rib cage and move with this swing if you consider just one of your legs at a time. I suggest you start on a circle line in either direction and focus on feeling the lift of your thigh on the outside of your horse when its inside leg steps under the body. This movement is more obvious than feeling your inside leg dipping down or in. Just as in the walk, in the sitting trot you can teach yourself to feel when each hind leg steps under your horse's body. Then, your leg aid for either more reach or a lateral step can be timed for when your horse's leg is off the ground and can answer the aid. Your aids can become more subtle and accurate. Aids not applied in rhythm risk tension in your horse. Aids given in rhythm improve the chance that your horse answers correctly. Thoughtful aids help you work less physically by thinking more. Timing your aids correctly develops feel and harmony.

A discussion of sitting trot is not complete without considering the quality of the horse's trot. The better the horse's balance, connection, and engagement, the more the trot movement is taken in the horse's body, and not in the rider's body. There are many considerations, but all things being equal, to protect my back, I avoid sitting the trot on a given horse until it has attained a degree of suppleness and connection so that the trot is not jarring.

Consider "what moves and what shouldn't move much" at sitting trot. The lumbar spine is *not* a place to seek movement in the sitting trot. Doing so risks excess strain and wear and tear on the intervertebral joints and intervertebral disks. So, do not absorb the movement of the sitting trot in your back. This risks too much movement in the spine in an unhealthy way. A bit of pelvic lift in the up phase of the sitting trot is not a terrible strategy, but avoid spine extension, or arching, when your weight returns down onto your horse's back. This risks straining your spine. Again, it is too simple to say that your lumbar spine and pelvis do not move in sitting trot. Most certainly they do. There must be *some* movement in these joints. But, do not absorb the movement of the trot only in these joints. Rather, support the spine and pelvis as much as possible so the down forces of the sitting trot do not result in shear strain across the joints of your spine. Seeking balance and self-carriage, going up and forward in space with your horse, stabilizing your spine with your abdominal seat belt, and finding movement at your hip joints—joints meant to move—are more logical strategies. These strategies have helped riders who've come to me looking for ways to avoid back pain from riding. You can check if your spine alignment is stable at sitting trot by observing or feeling the rib-cage-to-pelvis distance at the front of your body. If this distance is steady, so is your spine alignment.

The challenge of sitting the trot often leads to shoulder tension, precluding suppleness in muscles of the shoulder and elbow. As a result, rather than a quiet hand position, your hands bounce up and down with the trot's movement. At the sitting trot, you must feel as if your arms become part of the bridle and your hands stay steady to your horse's mouth. This is tricky to feel. The movement at the shoulder and elbow that allows a stable hand position at both posting and sitting trot is very subtle. To clarify this skill, I teach riders to anchor their hands either by pressing their baby finger against either side of the horse's withers or looping their baby finger under a bucking strap. With hand position stabilized, the rider can then feel the movement necessary at the elbow during posting and sitting trot to accomplish steady contact with the horse. The bounce with dowel exercise develops this skill off horse.

My Challenge: Learning "What Moves and What Shouldn't Move Much" at Walk and Trot

Two horses helped me clarify my ideas about "what should move and what shouldn't move much" at walk and trot: Mac, my husband's mellow and veteran 15.2h Appaloosa gelding, and a similarly mellow Morgan gelding that I leased for my "riding rehab," after I recovered from back surgery.

On Mac, I spent time at walk feeling how his body moved and how I moved with it. I felt his swinging rib cage and struggled to link this movement with his steps. I'd ask myself which hind leg was stepping under his body. I'd speak a rhythm: right-left-right-left. Then I'd check to see if I was correct by looking at his shoulder. If I was incorrect, I'd watch his shoulder or his croup and visually determine when his hind legs were swinging under his body. I'd put in my head the correct "right-left-right-left" stepping and then feel what my body was doing. In this way I could correctly link the movement of my body with his. From this came the images I offer in this book of how to feel when each hind leg steps under your horse's body at walk and trot.

I practiced sitting trot on the Morgan, a more schooled dressage horse. By this time I knew that maintaining proper alignment was absolutely key to preserving what I had left of my spine and preventing further damage. I was determined to figure out how to do this. This horse had a reasonable trot to sit and was reliable enough for me to practice sitting trot with one hand on the reins. I placed my other hand on the front of my body as a pair of calipers, measuring the distance between my ribs and pelvis, and figured out how to keep this distance stable, and, hence, my spine stable, during sitting trot. With practice came the "seat belt" tool, as well as awareness of the swing of the horse's rib cage, and my legs at the hip joints.

Bounce with dowel

This exercise refines your ability to keep your hands steady when you are moving up and down, a skill needed for trot work.

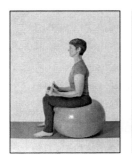 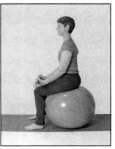 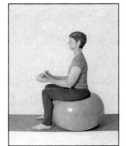 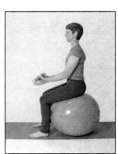

| *Photo 5-11* | *Photo 5-12* | *Photo 5-13* | *Photo 5-14* |

1. Sit on an exercise ball in neutral spine alignment.

2. Hold a 3-foot dowel or stick (a riding crop or whip will do) in your hands out in front of you, elbows bent by your sides (Photo 5-11).

3. Start bouncing on the ball. You will see that the dowel bounces up and down with you.

4. Now rest your hands and dowel on your knees. Bounce again (Photo 5-12). You will notice that since your knees are not going up and down, the dowel position stays stable, and your elbow joints move as you bounce. This is the feeling you are after when riding either the posting or sitting trot. Your hands stay still while your body goes up and down.

5. Lift your hands off your legs so they are again in the air holding the dowel (Photo 5-13).

6. Now, as you bounce, try to keep your hands and the dowel still in space (Photo 5-14).

Keeping your hands and the dowel still in space while your body bounces up and down requires awareness and movement at the elbow joint. If this is too hard, have someone hold the dowel still to help you feel the subtle movement at your elbow joint. Alternately tighten your arm muscles so the dowel (and your hands) bounce with you, and then release these muscles so the dowel stays still while you bounce; your elbow joints move to allow stillness of your hands and the dowel.

The Rider's Challenge: Unstable Spine at Sitting Trot
Rebecca and Tipper

Remember Rebecca? (See "The Rider's Challenge: Unstable Spine at Posting Trot" in this chapter.) This enthusiastic high school student had some challenges maintaining stability of her long torso at the posting trot. Now we move on to the sitting trot.

I am not surprised to see Rebecca's spine move too much at sitting trot. Her tight leg and hip joint lock against Tipper's body, forcing movement into her spine. This gripping also puts her slightly out of synch with Tipper's rhythm; her "up and down" lags Tipper's "up and down."

I describe my four strategies for sitting the trot, emphasizing her self-carriage and abdominal seat belt support. I don't spend a lot of time telling Rebecca to not grip. To me it doesn't make sense to tell a muscle to release and "let go" when it has taken on the job of keeping you "safe" and stable in the saddle. Rather, I think of the muscles that should be working to keep you in the saddle (your core) and focus on them "doing more." Relaxing the gripping legs without finding a different strategy to stay in the saddle guarantees the gripping will quickly return.

Back on the rail, I have Rebecca think of lifting herself up out of the saddle with Tipper and carrying herself forward with him. This improves her ability to stay in synch with his trot. I also have her call out loud the 1-2-1-2 stepping of the hind legs. She finds this remarkably hard to do; her rhythm often falls behind Tipper's. But once she gets a more proactive approach to staying with Tipper at the trot, her spine stability improves.

Rebecca also needs a lot of help from her abdominal seat belt to support her spine. We review this tool and I encourage her to experiment with how much effort she needs for a more stable body. We again use her hand as a set of calipers on the front of her abdomen so she can feel if her rib-cage-to-pelvis distance changes much with each trot step.

Like many riders, Rebecca discovers that it is easier to feel the positive effect of her abdominal seat belt if her torso is tipped slightly behind the vertical. This helps her feel the horse move out in front of her stable body position. Ideally in the end, her body will be closer to the vertical, but for now this helps her support her spine. We also start at a relatively slow trot.

After a few rounds of focusing on counting the trot steps and keeping her abdominal seat belt on, her gripping legs begin to release, allowing her thighbones to move with Tipper's barrel. I ask if she can feel this movement.

"Sort of," she answers. "They definitely feel looser than before."

I have Rebecca pick up a circle to the right and settle into a steady rhythm. I coach her to feel her left (outside) thigh lift up as I call out "now" when Tipper's right (inside) hind leg steps forward under his body. From her core stability, and the cue "now" in rhythm with the trot, she can feel how her legs move with Tipper's body. Gradually Tipper's trot becomes freer and covers more ground as Rebecca's gripping legs release and allow Tipper's back to swing. And, Rebecca enjoys improved spine stability and hip-joint muscle suppleness. Now she is moving with Tipper—and smiling.

Exercises for Rebecca: Bounce in rhythm 1-4, abdominal curls, plank on mat—knees and feet, plank on ball, quadruped—single and diagonal, knee circles, leg circles, leg lifts on ball

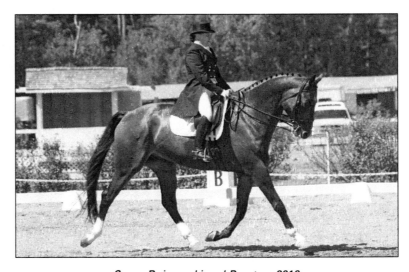

Caryn Bujnowski and Preston, 2010.

Here is a riding exercise to help you improve your connection with your horse at sitting trot and explore how attention to your body facilitates your horse's movement.

- Establish a circle right at sitting trot. The size can depend upon your level of training, but 15 to 20 meters works well.

- Establish the tempo of your horse's trot in your head by counting the stepping of the hind legs: 1-2-1-2, etc.

- Change the 1 and 2 to right and left, matching the hind leg that is stepping under your horse's body. Try to identify which hind leg steps under the body by feeling how your thighbones move at the hip joint. Recall that your outside thighbone will lift up as your horse's inside hind leg steps under its body. If you aren't sure of the stepping of your horse's hind legs, simply watch its shoulders. Like learning your posting diagonals, the opposite shoulder will come forward with the hind leg in question.

- Add rhythmic emphasis on the stepping under of the inside (in this case, the right) hind leg: *right*-left-*right*-left-*right*-left, and so on. Feel how your body moves with this rhythm. Feel that both your inside, or right thigh, dips down, and your outside, or left thigh, lifts up when you say "right." This helps your inside leg support your horse's engaging inside-right hind leg, and helps your outside thigh allow the outward swing of the rib cage. Both help your horse maintain bend and rhythm.

- Practice this exercise in both directions, emphasizing the inside or *left* hind leg when tracking left.

- Finally, establish a figure of eight movement with two equally sized circles of 15 to 20 meters. Find the rhythm as described above. Now you will have to change the emphasis of your right-left metronome as you change direction. This is challenging.

- As you change direction in the figure of eight, switch from *right*-left-*right*-left to *left*-right-*left*-right—again, the emphasis is on the inside hind leg as it reaches under your horse's body. It may take a few steps for you to make the change in emphasis. With practice you can do it quickly, and develop the skill to support the bend and rhythm of your horse's trot in any direction or change of direction. This skill translates into riding the hind legs appropriately in lateral work.

The Rider's Challenge: Unsteady Hands at Trot
Tamara and Jake

Tamara is a petite novice rider well matched to her 15h Arab gelding, Jake. Like many adult riders, she started riding as a kid, and then stopped for school, career, and family. She is motivated to improve her riding as much as possible within her restricted riding schedule.

Tamara and Jake are warming up when I arrive. I watch for a few minutes as they do some walk and trot work. Jake is a willing worker but can be fussy in the contact. Tamara has decent balance but does not always have control of her arms and at times conveys a disorganized picture. I note particularly that Tamara's arms move a lot during the posting trot. This is where we start.

Tamara and Jake proceed at walk, and I help Tamara feel Jake's rhythm, rib cage swing, and, particularly, how his head and neck move at the walk. At trot, the energy from Jake's body causes Tamara's shoulders to tighten. As a result, her arms lock and post up and down with her body. Rather than having a stable contact with Jake through the bridle, her hands are moving. I have Tamara reach both of her baby fingers down to Jake's withers so they have a reference point. Then, as Tamara moves off in posting trot, by keeping her hands contacting Jake's body, she begins to feel what it is like for her body, but not her hands, to move up and down in the posting trot. This requires shoulder and elbow suppleness not initially possible because of tension.

We practice several rounds of posting trot in both directions. At times Tamara succeeds in stabilizing her hands by moving her elbow joints. I give Tamara two images: One is to feel her body swing through her arms; the other is to imagine a tray resting on her forearms. These images help her focus on her body movement and arm stability.

As expected, the sitting trot presents the same problem. Tamara tries not to bounce, and her shoulders tense up around her ears. Her hands bounce with her body with the expected annoyance from Jake, who hollows and moves forward reluctantly.

I review sitting trot strategies with Tamara, emphasizing the abdominal seat belt for security. After a few circles of alternating sitting and posting trot, she isn't quite as stiff, but her hands are still unstable. I again have her rest her hands on Jake's neck for stability and clarity of position. She keeps her hands stable for just a few steps of sitting trot before her shoulder tension returns, pulling Tamara's hands away from Jake's neck.

I advise Tamara to practice a stable hand position at posting trot before working at sitting trot. She begins by doing just a few steps of sitting trot at a time, either by alternating between posting and sitting, or coming to walk. Over time, with improved core stability and awareness, she achieves more control of her arms and hands.

Exercises for Tamara: Plank on ball, plank on mat—knees and feet, leg lifts on ball, hug-a-tree—both arms and single arm, bounce with dowel

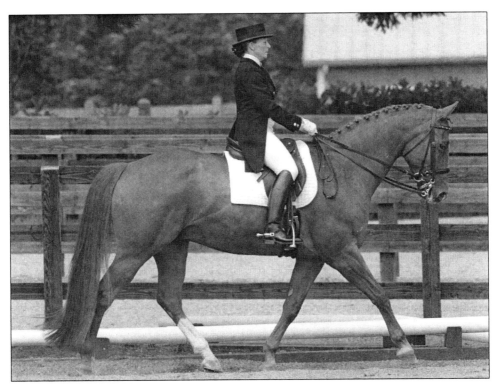

Mary Houghton and W. King's Ransom, 2010.

Canter

The canter is a three-beat gait with a moment of suspension, as shown in Figure 5-3. For the right lead, the order of footfall is LH, RH and LF together, RF, moment of suspension. Unlike the walk and trot in which the hind legs move in opposition to each other, in the canter the hind legs initially move almost together during the first two beats of the gait. This results in an undulating, or rolling, path of energy through the horse's back, from the outside hind leg to the inside foreleg.

To find the canter rhythm, focus on the swinging of the hind legs under your horse's body. Think of it as one large beat and say in your head "*can* ter, *can* ter, *can* ter," with the emphasis on the two hind legs swinging under. This emphasis informs the timing of the driving aids: when needed, they should occur on the first beat (*can*) when the hind legs are swinging under your horse's body and can respond.

Canter: What moves and what shouldn't move much
- Your arms follow the motion of your horse's head and neck.
- Your legs are stable.
- Your hip joints allow the rolling back-to-front motion of your horse's body, especially your inside hip joint.
- Your torso stays in correct alignment, without excess rocking forward and back. The more collected the canter, the less your torso rocks; it adopts a more up-and-down motion with your horse.

I have found the canter to be the most variable gait among horses, and struggle, quite frankly, to find a concrete answer to the question we've asked for each gait: what moves and what shouldn't move much? As discussed, your arms must allow your horse's head and neck to move. And, although your legs should be stable, they can only be still if you have enough suppleness in your hip joint muscles to allow the undulation of your horse's body to move through this joint. Think of your balanced torso riding the canter much like a bobbing cork or float riding the upward energy of a wave. The float stays on top of the wave and is not disturbed, from a balance standpoint, by the wave. In the same way, you should feel upright on your horse.

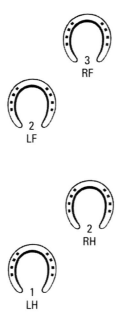

Figure 5-3. Canter footfall diagram, right lead.

The nature of your horse's movement at canter encourages your body to move front to back. It is easy for the horse's movement to send your body forward too much—as your horse's hind legs step under and its forehand comes up—and then send your body backward too much, behind the vertical, when it comes down on its leading foreleg. Some of this motion is appropriate, but it should not be exaggerated. Also, any torso movement should preserve neutral spine alignment; the movement should happen at the hip joint, not at the intervertebral joints.

Lateral balance can become quite problematic at the canter. When cantering in a circle, it is challenging to sit in the middle of your horse when the side upon which you tend to sit heavily is on the outside of the circle. It is as if centrifugal force from the canter throws you to the outside. Unfortunately this unbalances your horse and makes clear aids difficult. Practice establishing lateral balance and symmetry at walk and trot before expecting great things at the canter. And remember, just because it feels odd does *not* mean that it is wrong. Let your horse be your guide and check your position. If your horse tends to fall on its outside shoulder at canter in one direction, check that you are not falling to the outside of the saddle on that side, contributing to the imbalance.

The Rider's Challenge: Stiff Arms and Legs at Canter
Kim and Oswald

Kim is a studious intermediate rider who is always looking for ways to improve her riding. "I feel I need to work hard to keep him going, especially in the canter," she tells me.

I watch Kim ride her 8-year-old 2nd level Swedish gelding, Oswald. Overall she has a positive focus, and a fairly correct and strong posture. Her arm and leg positions look a bit forced, as if she works to keep them in place. When I see this, I always go back and reevaluate posture.

I get some ideas for improving Kim's riding efficiency (helping her *think* more and *work* less) at canter. To my eye, her arms are quite still, while her upper back, hinging at her waist, presses back in an exaggerated motion as Oswald canters onto his leading foreleg. At the same time, by necessity, there is more arch, or extension, in Kim's lumbar spine. Kim's hip angle remains fixed.

Kim demonstrates a common scenario at canter: her hip and shoulder joint muscles lack suppleness. This is manifest by an exaggerated torso rocking that results in spine alignment changes.

Three things need to happen to improve Kim's function at canter. First, her arms must allow movement of the horse's head and neck. At halt, I have Kim move her arms forward and back, in line with the bit, to help her appreciate the range of motion the arms can have, and the movement possible at the elbow and shoulder joints. Second, her hip joint must be less locked so that the canter movement can pass through the joint with less disruption of posture. This, of course, can only happen with a more secure understanding of correct posture, which leads to the third challenge: correct postural support. Kim's upper back and body need to stay balanced over her pelvis. For this I explain the same planes image that I used for Jennifer (see "The Rider's Challenge: S-Shaped Posture" in Chapter 2). That is, imagine the upper back in the area of the shoulder blades as one plane, and the abdominal wall as another plane. The upper back plane needs to press forward at the same time the abdominal wall plane presses back. These actions decrease the excess upper back rounding and lumbar spine extension Kim adopts during the canter.

Kim bravely experiments first with moving her arms more and letting her legs rest heavily on the stirrup with less gripping. At first she exaggerates her arm movement, which I think is a good thing. She hones in on an amount of movement that allows a steady contact with Oswald. With improved arm suppleness, she improves her posture by bringing both her upper back plane and her lower abdominal plane toward the middle of her body. Improved posture allows improved movement in her hip joints. Amazingly, Oswald bounds more freely upward and forward in the canter. Horses are so sensitive! A seemingly small change in how Kim organizes her body makes a world of difference in his way of going.

Exercises for Kim: Plank on ball, plank on mat—knees and feet, knee circles, leg circles, partner arm suppleness

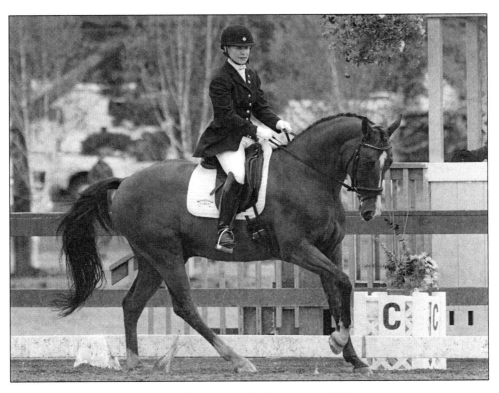

Paula Helm and H.S. Whrapsody, 2010.

The Rider's Challenge: Pumping Gluteal Muscles at Canter
Sheila and Jade

Sheila is a novice adult rider proud to have mastered walk and trot on her 10-year-old Fjord mare, Jade. She now wants to improve their canter.

I watch Sheila and Jade work first at walk and trot. Sheila tends to push with her gluteal muscles at both walk and trot, so when she tries a canter depart with Jade, she uses the same strategy, pumping the pelvis into a tuck with her glutes, to keep Jade going. The problem is, however, the harder she pumps, the more Jade hollows, breaking from the canter into a fast and bouncy trot.

I explain to Sheila that her overworking gluteal muscles are working against her. I start by showing Sheila how much she is using her gluteal muscles at walk and trot. I show her how to focus on using just her lower leg for a driving aid and less of her gluteal muscles (just as I did for Linda and Wendberg; see "The Rider's Challenge: Overusing the Gluteal Muscles" in Chapter 2). This requires Sheila to maintain her position in the saddle by not letting her leg grip or gluteal muscles tighten. To help her gain awareness of her gluteal muscles tightening, at halt, I have her squeeze them tightly, and then release them.

Back in the canter, I coach Sheila to again use her lower leg as an aid. She struggles with this, as her leg tends to cling to Jade's side in the canter. Without her legs free to give a "go" aid, she is left using her pelvis to try and keep the canter, which is not successful, and Jade falls into a trot.

I coach Sheila in a sitting trot to help her feel her abdominal seat belt stabilize her pelvis to the back of the saddle and to help her feel more secure in her position and balance. This allows her gripping legs to let go. We then go back into canter, and I encourage her to feel her pelvis stay relatively still in the saddle while her legs remain free to aid Jade. We review leg aid timing: her legs encourage Jade to canter as the hind legs sweep under Jade's body. I coach Sheila to add a rhythmic tap with her whip if Jade doesn't answer her leg aid. This prevents Sheila from pumping and gripping if Jade doesn't respond to just the lower leg. I have her feel herself going up and forward with Jade in the canter.

These images and tools help Sheila avoid gripping and pumping with her gluteal muscles, and as a result, Jade canters more easily. She quickly is on a positive feedback loop of less pumping, more canter, even less pumping and looser legs, rhythmic leg aids, and a canter that is much easier to maintain.

Exercises for Sheila: Pelvic bridge—simple and single leg, knee circles, leg circles, leg lifts on ball

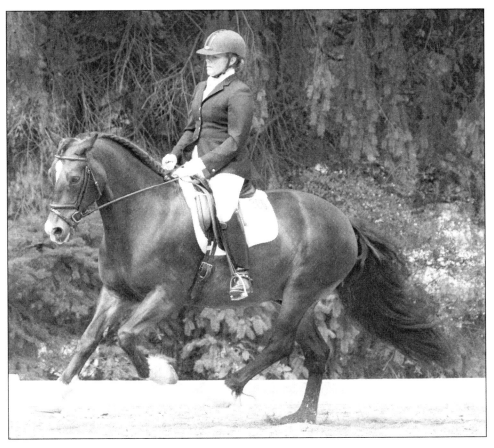

Lisa Boyer and Winterlake Gulliver (owned by Yvonne Billera), 2010.

Transitions

Transitions are immensely beneficial for developing balance and self-carriage in your horse and are a fundamental check of your horse's training progress. But remember: you are a part of that team. What can you do to enable your horse to do a balanced transition and not create problems?

There are two components of a transition to consider: rhythm and energy. A transition may involve a change in rhythm and/or a change in energy. For example, riding a transition from a working trot to a trot lengthening does not involve a rhythm change, but it does involve a change (an increase) in energy. Riding a trot-to-walk transition involves a change in rhythm (trot rhythm to walk rhythm) and a change (decrease) in energy. Some transitions are tricky, and we could quibble about how to characterize them. For example, is there a change in rhythm or energy going from collected trot to medium trot? The rhythm stays the same. I say there is an increase in energy, but the change is more in how the horse *uses* the energy. For collection, the energy is sent more upward, and for the medium trot, it is sent both up and out. The canter-to-trot transition is also interesting. It is a difficult transition with a clear change in rhythm. I would argue, however, that usually there isn't much of a change in energy—the horse doesn't really slow down going from canter to trot. In fact, slowing the horse down to get from canter to trot impairs the subsequent trot quality.

Regardless of which transition components are most important, you must be ready for the change in your body—in energy and rhythm—and prepare to move appropriately with your horse. This takes focus, postural support, and body control. With organization, you will maximize the benefit of transitions on your horse's balance and make them look effortless and harmonious.

Upward Transitions

In all transitions, you must stay balanced—despite the change in your horse's energy—and move appropriately with the ensuing gait. In up transitions, the energy increases. To ride a balanced up transition, anticipate the increased forward energy and avoid being left behind. Establish a proactive mind-set, self-carriage from core balance, and a "come with me" intent to encourage the increased energy from your horse. Your leg aids provide the final cues for the up transitions; be ready to move in the rhythm of the new gait.

Downward Transitions

Just as in the up transitions, maintaining balance is key for a good-quality down transition. Without preparation, a down transition can cause you to fall forward. Most downward transitions result in less forward energy. Use your core muscles to prepare your body for that decreased energy. I think of the front of the body functioning like a wall that tells the horse, "I'm not going forward so much anymore, and neither should you." Basing the down transitions with the intent of your body assists your balance and prevents an abrupt restricting rein aid. As in the up transition, be prepared to move in the rhythm of the new gait.

A common error in riding down transitions is positioning your body behind the vertical and leaning back, using body weight at times against the reins to facilitate the transition. While appropriate in a bolting runaway horse, it is not appropriate in horse training. Leaning back does not encourage your horse to step underneath you from behind, raise its back, or gain better balance off its forehand. Rather, leaning back encourages your horse to fall on its forehand. In a halt or down transition, if your horse is strong in the bridle, seek strong stability from your torso against the pulling rein and use carefully timed driving aids (legs and intent) to guide the horse to step under itself in better self-carriage. Bending lines and lateral steps help guide the horse to better balance. Horse training aside, however, it's important that you not let your horse's poor balance change *you*. If you do, you've given your horse the green light to do it again—your horse changed your posture and balance, hence its strategy has been reinforced. You remain effective only when you keep a stable body position despite your horse's actions, reactions, and balance challenges.

Specific Transitions
Walk-to-Halt or Trot-to-Halt Transition

Consider what happens when going from either walk or trot to a halt. You go from moving with your horse as appropriate for the given gait, to not moving at all. That is the basis of your halt aid. Stop moving. Breathe to facilitate this transition. For walk to halt, note that your arms and legs are moving with your horse, and your pelvis moves somewhat too. Take an inhale breath, and as you exhale, firm up your core muscles to stabilize your pelvis and anchor your arms by your sides. You needn't pull back to accomplish this transition: simply stop your movement. The same strategy will work for trot to halt. Your horse will quickly learn this aid. Done this way, the halt aid happens without pulling and promotes balance and harmony. You appear as if you've done "nothing." But in fact, you've ridden the transition in a thoughtful, organized, balanced, and logical manner. This makes it look easy.

Trot-to-Walk Transition

Focus on the change of rhythm that happens going from trot to walk. As you do with other transitions, use your breath to organize and center, and then add a bit more tone to give that "don't go forward so much" message to your horse. Be prepared to soften your aid as soon as your horse walks so you do not lose energy. Often this transition results in a loss of forward energy—your horse abruptly props itself on its forelegs and then needs to reorganize into the walk.

Try this exercise to improve your trot-to-walk transition:

- Establish an active trot, either posting or sitting.
- Initiate the transition to walk not by pulling on the reins, but by slowing how your body moves with your horse—slow your posting or sitting rhythm. Use Pilates breathing to balance and encourage stability and integrity of your body so your horse can hear your change in tempo.
- Keep gradually slowing your tempo until your horse comes to a walk. You should find that in the resulting walk, your horse moves forward freely.

It may take many trot steps to accomplish the walk transition at first. But, over time, your horse will learn the "don't go forward so much" cue from your body and breathing, and quickly come to a prompt, balanced, and active walk. The transition comes from managing your horse's energy from your center and steadying—not pulling on—the reins. This promotes balance and harmony between you and your horse.

Canter-to-Trot Transition

This is a very challenging transition to do well. For this transition, think of going from canter to trot as just a change in rhythm, with little or no change in energy. I use Pilates breathing to prepare (again, your half halt and the horse's half halt!). Give a short steadying squeeze with the outside rein, exhale, and stabilize your body into an imagined trot rhythm. Sometimes it takes several tries for your horse to understand the aids for this transition, but basing this transition in your center and focusing on the rhythm change has a beneficial balancing effect on your horse. It makes clear to both you and your horse what is changing. Simply pulling on the reins can result in slowing the canter and losing impulsion, causing your horse to fall into an unbalanced trot.

Canter-to-Walk Transition

This transition requires more skill in terms of timing. It makes most sense to ask for this transition when your horse's hind legs swing under its body, and it has a chance to balance on its haunches during the decline in forward motion. Prepare by feeling the canter rhythm. Earlier I described simplifying the canter rhythm to a two-beat count: *can* ter, *can* ter, with *can* being the time when your horse's hind legs swing under, and the *ter* part being when its forehand comes onto the leading foreleg. The aid for the canter-walk transition should come with the *can* to facilitate your horse coming to walk when it otherwise would come onto the leading foreleg. Ride the canter rhythm and use an exhale breath to say "don't go forward so much" and to stabilize and anchor your arms by your sides. Soften the rein aid when your horse walks.

Within Gait Transitions, Up and Down

Within gait transitions come from maintaining a steady tempo and rhythm (by understanding the horse's gait and using your mental metronome) and modulating the amount of forward versus upward energy. Your body directs the energy up for collection, up and out for medium gaits, and out for extended gaits. Imagine arrows in the middle of your body, one is directed upward (collection) and one is directed outward (extension). Within gait transitions emphasize one of these arrows in your body (Figure 5-4).

To do a down transition from medium trot to collected trot, for example, sit tall and use an exhale breath (this gives both you and your horse a half halt) to draw your core muscles inward and tell your horse not to go forward so much. At the same time, close your fingers on the reins but avoid being so strong in the bridle that your horse loses impulsion. Keep a pronounced rhythm in your body and your hip joints swinging in rhythm to keep your horse in trot, but one that doesn't cover so much ground. Be prepared to give a

leg aid or a tap with the whip to encourage your horse to step under into collected trot. For sure, you may find the need to give a driving aid in the down
transition from medium to collected trot so your horse does not lose activity.

To do an upward transition from collected trot to medium trot, with
your horse actively engaged and with you, send energy out in front of you
(Figure 5-4) with intent. Support a stable rhythm with your body to counteract your horse's tendency to trot with a quicker tempo rather than with
longer steps. Provide enough stability through the bridle to prevent your
horse from falling on its forehand. If your horse needs more forward energy
to accomplish the longer trot steps, apply your driving leg aids in rhythm,
stay balanced over the center of your horse, and, if needed, add a tapping of
the whip in rhythm with the gait. Many riders fall behind the vertical in trot
lengthenings, or medium or extended trot. This is not an efficient position,
however, because leaning back encourages your horse onto its forehand. As
well, this imperfect alignment requires you to compensate, either through
gripping legs or through a restraining rein. Better control comes from correct posture and spine alignment balanced over your horse, moving forward
with your horse.

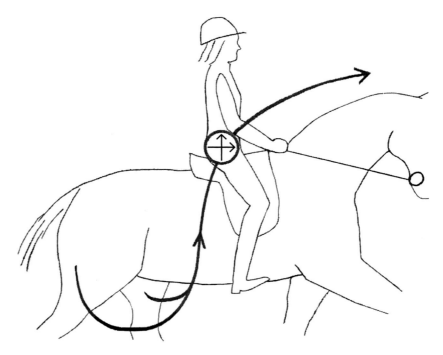

*Figure 5-4. This rider energy diagram shows how the rider, through her center,
can direct the horse in varied degrees of upward and forward.*

The Rider's Challenge: Balance during Transitions
Leslie and Sprinx

We earlier met Leslie and Sprinx (see "The Rider's Challenge: Tempo Control from Center" in this chapter), who struggle with balance and steadiness at the trot, and with balance in down transitions.

As Leslie and Sprinx work on gaining harmony and a steady trot, I notice that whenever Leslie comes to a walk or halt, balance is a real problem. When I cue her for a down transition, Leslie pushes her feet in front of her and leans back against the reins. The resulting transition is abrupt and on the forehand, with Sprinx propping against her front legs. I wait to work on transitions until Leslie understands the power she has over Sprinx by riding from her center, rather than riding from her feet and hands.

I first have Leslie try walk-to-halt transitions using her breath and avoiding a change in her body position—that is, keeping her feet underneath her and not leaning back.

Leslie is skeptical, but gives it a try. On the first few attempts Sprinx wanders a bit. Leslie struggles to not buy into Sprinx's wandering by leaning back and pulling. After three or four tries, however, Leslie feels how simplifying her transition aids from "moving with Sprinx" to "not moving with Sprinx" results in a better balanced and less abrupt halt. Sprinx begins to focus more on Leslie, cocking her ears back in anticipation of the next cue.

Adjusting Leslie's strategies for riding trot-to-walk transitions is more challenging. Back in posting trot, I again guide Leslie to good spine alignment with her feet underneath her. I have her ride a walk transition by slowing her posting until Sprinx walks.

I clarify to Leslie that in the end, I am not after a trot-to-walk transition that takes many slowing trot steps, but Leslie can feel that when she rides the transition to walk by slowing the trot, Sprinx does not lose balance and forward direction in the resulting walk. Leslie is forced to keep her balance because she is posting, and Sprinx is forced to keep her balance because Leslie does not offer a rein for her to lean on. The walk that results is forward and active.

I assure Leslie that with practice she will not have to take so much time to get from trot to walk. But done this way, she learns to use her center as the basis of the trot-to-walk transition, rather than pressing into her feet and leaning back against the reins. And Sprinx will learn to listen to Leslie's center and come to walk in better balance, rather than propping against her front legs. The resulting walk will have better energy, and Leslie and Sprinx will stay in balance and harmony.

Exercises for Leslie: Bounce in rhythm 1-4, abdominal curls, crisscross, plank on mat—knees and feet, plank on ball, leg lifts on ball

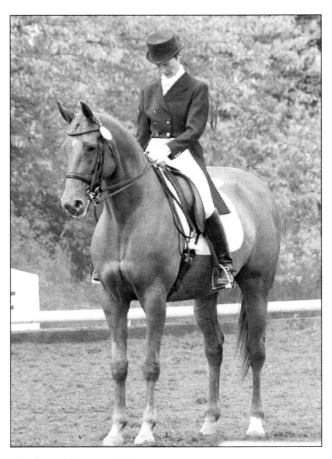

Beth and Bluette, 2003 (copyright 2007 Scarlett Pflugrad, Edmonds, WA).

Lateral Movements

The Rider Checklist is put to full use tackling the lateral movements, including leg yield, shoulder-in, travers, and half pass. Focus on the movement at hand: be sure you know what you are asking for from your horse! Keep precise balance so you can guide your horse sideways. Control the arm and leg aids so they do not put you off balance—this can be challenging. Finally, appropriately time your aids with the rhythm of your horse. It is beyond the scope of this book to discuss the details of every lateral movement; I have some general thoughts and will use the leg yield as an example.

Some advise you to sit *heavily* on the seat bone in the direction of travel to accomplish lateral work. I fear this can disrupt balance in both you and your horse. A dramatic shift in your weight can cause your horse to fall, rather than to carry itself, in the direction of travel. This advice also risks your twisting out of correct alignment. I suggest that you sit *to* the direction of travel, keeping your pelvis level. For example, if you are doing a leg yield to the right, sit to the right as if you are creating a tiny space that will allow your horse room to move to the right underneath you. This allows you to stay balanced, align your shoulders over your pelvis, and shift toward the direction of travel. By keeping your pelvis balanced (not heavily weighted on one side), you preserve body alignment and are more likely to have equal access to both rein and legs aids to precisely direct your horse's energy. In the energy diagram with *upward* and *forward* arrows (Figure 5-4), add an arrow directing the horse to the side, and send your energy along that line.

The leg yield is a great exercise to practice working with your horse's gaits and applying aids at a logical time to improve your horse's response. It helps you and your horse move together. The example below describes the aids of a leg yield to the left, with your horse moving away from your right leg. I'll describe doing the leg yield from the quarter line of the arena to the arena wall.

- Turn down the quarter line on the right rein. Establish a straight line with an active trot.
- Feel the right-left stepping of your horse's hind legs.
- When the right leg steps under, add extra movement or swing of your right leg inward to direct the right hind leg to cross in front of the left hind leg.
- Keep your left rein supporting so your horse doesn't fall out the left shoulder.

- Be sure to keep a ground-covering trot during the exercise, with your mental metronome ticking away, "1-2-1-2," or even better, "right-left-right-left."
- During the lateral movement, however, change the words for the mental metronome to "over" (for the right hind leg) and "forward" (for the left hind leg): "over-forward-over-forward." In this way impulsion is maintained, and the lateral aid from your right leg occurs when your horse can respond (right hind leg in the air).
- Sit in the direction of travel without leaning or twisting. In this leg yield to the left, imagine your torso, balanced and aligned, going both forward and a bit to the left, as if making room, or a space, underneath the left side of your body for your horse to move into.

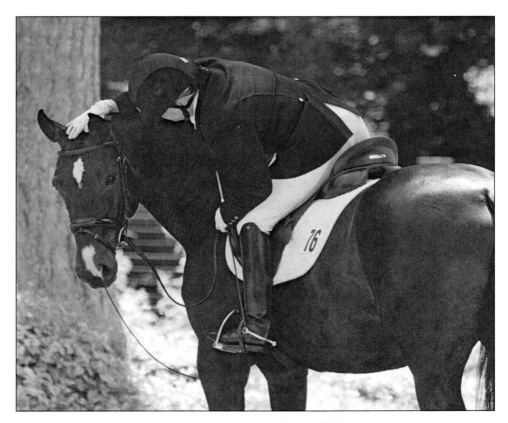

Caryn Bujnowski and Dylan, 2010.

Final Comments

Balanced riding = efficient riding = beautiful riding = harmonious riding

There are many details to keep track of while riding, and it is easy to think only about what your horse is doing. You owe it to your horse to also consider yourself, to always ask if your position and balance strategies are either causing or contributing to a training problem. With every step ask, "Where am I? Where is my body? Am I balanced? Am I moving with the gait?" After all, *you* are the cognitive member of the horse-rider pair, equipped with the analytical capabilities to solve problems. Be sure to include yourself as a potential part of a training problem, and use the Rider Checklist to assess your contribution to the problem and find solutions. As you develop these skills, you will be able to communicate with light aids and progress toward a wonderful state of balance and harmony with your horse.

You are the cognitive member of the horse-rider pair, equipped with the analytical capabilities to solve problems.

Suggested Workouts

Here are workout routines from exercises in this book.

Preride Warm-Up

Before you ride, take about ten minutes to organize your body with this sequence of exercises. These movements can be done on a chair or a bale of hay, instead of a ball. So you can do them in your barn before you ride. This sequence is designed to remind you of your body tools to improve your balance, awareness, and function before you get in the saddle.

- Pilates breathing 2 (use your hands on your torso rather than a stretchy band)

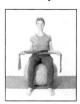

- Pelvic rocking on ball, front to back

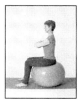

- Pelvic rocking on ball, side to side

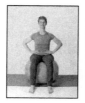 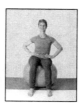

- Spine stretch forward, alternating with spine extension—scarecrow

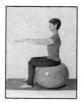 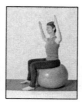

- Spine twist on ball

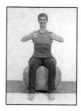 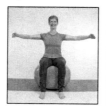 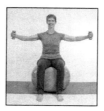

- Hug-a-tree—both arms

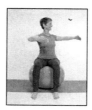 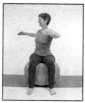

- Hug-a-tree—single arm

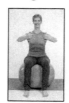

- Chest expansion

- Leg lifts on ball

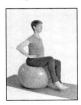

- Deep rotator, piriformis stretch—sitting

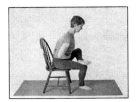

- Hamstring stretch—standing

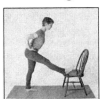

Basic Workout

Here are the easier versions of the exercises described in this book. With this workout, you will develop the skills and body tools described in the Rider Checklist: focus, posture, leg control, and arm control. Plus, the beginning bouncing sequence hones your ability to maintain a steady tempo and warms up your body.

On-the-ball warm-up

- Bounce in rhythm 1

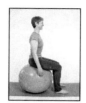

- Bounce in rhythm 2—arm swings

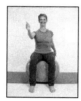

- Bounce in rhythm 4—ball jacks

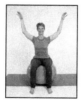 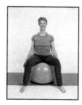 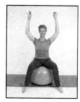

On-the-ball spine awareness warm-up

- Pilates breathing 2

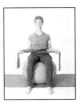

- Pelvic rocking on ball, front to back

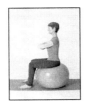 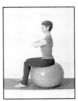

- Pelvic rocking on ball, side to side

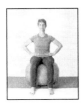

- Spine stretch forward, alternating with spine extension—scarecrow

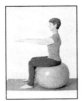 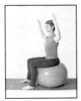 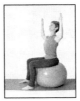

- Spine twist on ball

  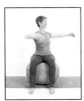

On-the-mat core work

- Abdominal curls

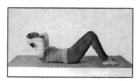

- Crisscross

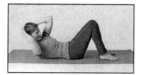

- Spine extension on mat

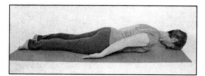 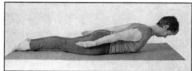

- Back stretch

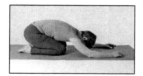

- Plank on mat—knees

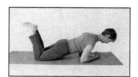

- Side planks—knees

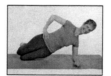

- Quadruped—single

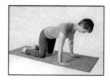 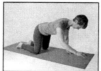 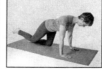

On-the-mat leg work

- Knee circles

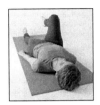 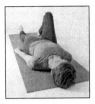

- Pelvic bridge—simple

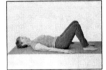 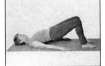

- Pelvic bridge—single leg

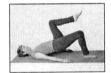

- Deep rotator, piriformis stretch

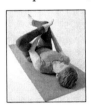

- Ball tongs—squeezes (on right)

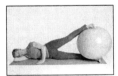 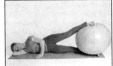

- Straight legs

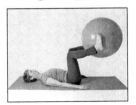 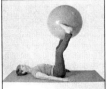

- Ball tongs—squeezes (on left)

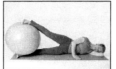

On-the-ball arm work
- Hug-a-tree—both arms

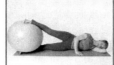

- Chest expansion

- Shoulder stretch

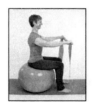

On-the-mat leg stretches
- Hip flexor stretch

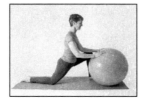

• Hamstring stretch (right)

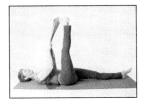

• Abductor stretch (right)

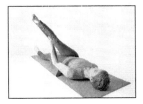

• Hamstring stretch (left)

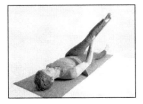

• Abductor stretch (left)

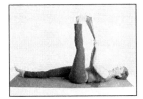

• Adductor stretch

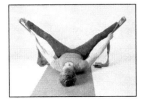

Intermediate Workout

This sequence of exercises is the more challenging version of the exercises described in this book. The workout further develops the skills and body tools of focus, posture, leg control, and arm control. If any exercise is too challenging for you, replace it with the simpler version from the Basic Workout (above). Remember, when you are fatigued, you risk losing form, precision, and balance. It is better to keep great alignment and focus than to struggle with an exercise.

On-the-ball warm-up

- Bounce in rhythm 1

- Bounce in rhythm 2—arm swings

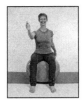

- Bounce in rhythm 3—toe tapping

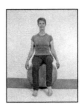

- Bounce in rhythm 4—ball jacks, including single arm and single leg variations

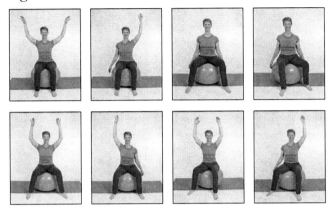

On-the-ball spine awareness warm-up

- Pilates breathing 2

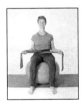

- Pelvic rocking on ball, front to back

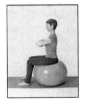

- Pelvic rocking on ball, side to side

- Spine stretch forward, alternating with spine extension—scarecrow

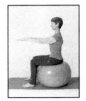

- Spine twist on ball

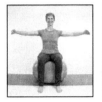

On-the-mat core work

- Abdominal curls sustained

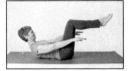 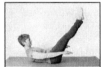

- Crisscross sustained

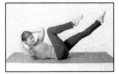 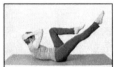

- Spine extension on mat

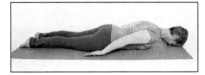 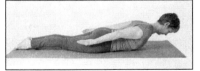

- Back stretch

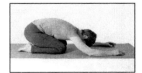

- Plank on mat—feet

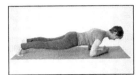

- Side planks—feet

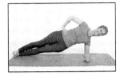

- Quadruped—diagonal

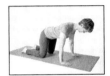 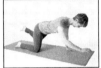

On-the-mat leg work

- Leg circles

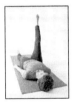

- Pelvic bridge with ball

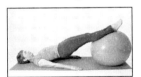

- Pelvic bridge with ball—balance

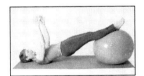

- Pelvic bridge with ball—single leg

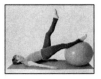

- Deep rotator, piriformis stretch

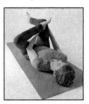

- Ball tongs—squeezes (on right without supporting left hand)

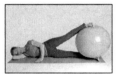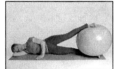

- Ball tongs—lifts (on right)

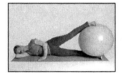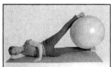

- Straight legs

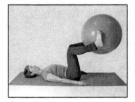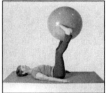

- Ball tongs—squeezes (on left without supporting right hand)

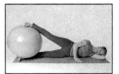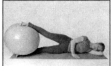

- Ball tongs—lifts (on left)

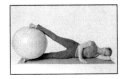 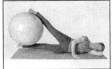

On-the-ball arm work

- Hug-a-tree—both arms

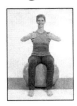 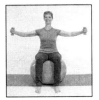

- Hug-a-tree—single arm

  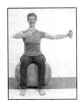

- Chest expansion

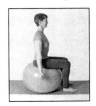

- Shoulder stretch

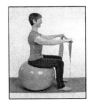

On-the-mat leg stretches

- Hip flexor stretch

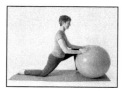

- Hamstring stretch (right)

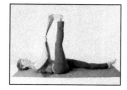

- Abductor stretch (right)

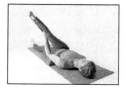

- Hamstring stretch (left)

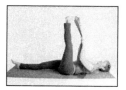

- Abductor stretch (left)

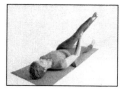

- Adductor stretch

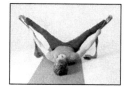

Glossary

Abduction. Movement of a body part away from the center of the body.

Adduction. Movement of a body part toward the center of the body.

Anterior. Facing toward or located in the front.

ASIS (Anterior Superior Iliac Spine). The prominent part of your pelvis just below your waist, sometimes referred to as your hip bone.

Balance. A state of bodily equilibrium. Balance is a condition of stability produced by even distribution of weight on each side of a vertical axis.

Bones. Form the rigid structure of the human skeleton. Bones are the levers that muscles move. Bones are connected with ligaments across joints.

Eversion. Refers to the ankle joint and involves both abduction and dorsiflexion and results in the bottom of the foot facing away from the center of the body.

Extension. In general, a movement at a joint that increases joint angle. From the anatomical position (standing, forward facing, arms by your sides, palms facing forward), extension of a limb brings it behind you. Therefore, extension of your spine results in bending backward, and extension of your hip joint brings your leg behind your body. An exception to this terminology is the ankle joint: extension of the ankle, or pointing the toe, is called plantar flexion (flexion of the ankle is called dorsiflexion).

Flexion. In general, a movement at a joint that decreases joint angle. From the anatomical position (standing, forward facing, arms by your sides, palms facing forward), flexing a limb brings it in front of you. Therefore, spine flexion results in bending forward. The exception is the knee: flexion of your knee, while it decreases joint angle, moves your lower leg behind you.

Focus. Keen attention to the job at hand.

Harmony. Cooperation and good communication. This is accomplished on horseback when you have good balance and aid timing so your horse can clearly hear you. Proper training of your horse assures that it responds to the aids. Good communication is then possible.

Inversion. Refers to the ankle joint; involves both adduction and plantar flexion and results in the bottom of the foot facing toward the center of the body.

Joint. Links bones together. Some joint configurations include a hinge joint (elbow joint and knee joint), and ball and socket joint (hip joint and shoulder joint). Joints are made of fibrous connective tissue and cartilage, and are supported by ligaments.

Loin. Some texts make reference to the rider's loins. Wikipedia defines this body part as the side of the human body between ribs and pelvis, or refers in general to the area below the ribs, or the general lower part of the body. This word has also been used to refer to genitals (hence the derivation of the term loincloth). Loin is not an anatomical term used in medicine, so I do not use it in this book.

Muscle. The contractile elements that move bones in relationship to each other. Muscles act by getting shorter and pulling—muscles do not push. The movement of bones in many directions results from muscles pulling in different directions. Muscles connect to bones via tendons.

Neutral spine alignment. Alignment of the spine such that its normal curves are present. When lying supine, neutral pelvic alignment is defined by the pubic bone and right and left ASIS being in a plane parallel to the floor.

Posterior. Facing toward or located in the back.

Posture. Alignment of the spine.

Relaxation. Mental or physical lack of tension. Relaxation is not a word I apply to riding. The mental component is not a trait I recommend while riding—a rider should be paying attention! Focus is a better word. Physical muscle relaxation is not what we seek while riding, but rather a cooperative tone that supports a stable position in motion. Relaxation is often used when *balance* and *suppleness* are more suitable. Muscle efficiency and organization, not relaxation, creates beautiful and graceful movement.

Rotation. Movement of the body in a horizontal plane. Rotation is either internal (toward the center of the body) or external (away from the center of the body).

Self-carriage. Responsible for one's own balance. For the rider, this means not relying on the reins for balance, and staying steady with the horse without gripping with the legs.

Supple. Just the right amount of muscle tone and effort at the right time, resulting in fluid and controlled movement. Supple movement is graceful movement.

Tension. Mental or physical lack of relaxation. Appropriate tension is needed to support upright posture on the moving horse. This tension should not be restrictive, but rather a coordinated muscle effort that creates stability.

Bibliography

Calais-Germain, Blandine. *Anatomy of Movement*. Seattle: Eastland Press, 1993.

Craig, Colleen. *Pilates on the Ball: The World's Most Popular Workout Using the Exercise Ball*. Rochester, VT: Healing Arts Press, 2001.

————. *Strength Training on the Ball: A Pilates Approach to Optimal Strength and Balance*. Rochester, VT: Healing Arts Press, 2005.

Crawford, Elizabeth. *Balance on the Ball: Exercises Inspired by the Teachings of Joseph Pilates*. San Francisco: Equilibrio, 2000.

Jenkins, David B. *Hollinshead's Functional Anatomy of the Limbs and Back*. 7th ed. Philadelphia: W.B. Saunders Company, 1998.

Lessen, Deborah, editor. *The PMA Pilates Certification Exam Study Guide*. Miami: Pilates Method Alliance, 2005.

Pilates, Joseph H. *Your Health: A Corrective System of Exercising that Revolutionizes the Entire Field of Physical Education*. 1934. Reprint, Incline Village, NV: Presentation Dynamics, Inc., 1998.

Pilates, Joseph H. Pilates, and William J. Miller. *Pilates' Return to Life Through Contrology*. 1945. Reprint, Incline Village, NV: Presentation Dynamics, Inc., 1998.

Richardson, Carolyn, Gwendolen Jull, Paul Hodges, Julie Hides. *Therapeutic Exercise for Spinal Segmental Stabilization in Low Back Pain: Scientific Basis and Clinical Approach*. London: Churchill Livingstone, 1999.

Index

Acknowledgments

I am grateful to my wonderful, thoughtful clients who asked questions that helped me clarify my ideas and urged me to forge ahead with this project.

This book would not have happened without the support of my husband, David Stutz. His calm trust was invaluable when my back injuries jeopardized my riding. He acknowledged my challenges and helped me stay patient and determined with my own healing and subsequent projects: training myself, developing my program, and writing it down in this book.

I thank my many equine partners, my most important teachers: Hematite, Travis, Talon, Mosby, Bluette, and Donner Girl. Thank you to Roxanne Christenson, Nancy Thacher, and the late Dietrich von Hopffgarten, for helping me with horse training over the years.

There are many people who gave me input over the course of this project. For reviewing the book, I thank Mary Bayley, Ann Shilling, Susan Miller, Janet Boggs, and Mary Cox. Endless encouragement to carry out this project came from my friends Perri Lynch and Jim Bennett; thank you for your support.

I am very grateful for the expert drawing skills of Sandy Johnson. Thank you to Courtney Secour for being my partner for the photographs of the partner exercises in the book. And thanks to Audrey Guidi for taking the time away from two young daughters to photograph the exercises. Thank you to Carolynn Bunch for her expert horse and rider photographs, and thank you to the riders willing to appear in the book.

It was a great pleasure to work with editor Karen Parkin, who carefully massaged my collection of ideas and stories into a very approachable and readable work. I so appreciate her patience and thoroughness, and willingness to answer my many questions. Thanks also go to Carolyn Acheson, indexer, and Janice Hussein, proofreader. Soundview Design then added their creative touch—it was so much fun to watch Amy Vaughn and David Marty blend the text, figures, and photos into a beautiful book.

About the Author

Beth Glosten, MD, created the RiderPilates program in Redmond, Washington, where she offers private Pilates sessions, small group exercise classes, and rider position-focused riding lessons. She also frequently travels to teach riding clinics that apply RiderPilates principles.

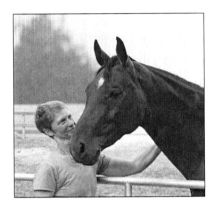

Beth received her Pilates training through the PhysicalMind Institute and is certified through the Pilates Method Alliance. She earned her medical degree from the University of Washington and had a career as an academic anesthesiologist, specializing in obstetric anesthesia. While she no longer practices medicine, her medical knowledge and experience inform her teaching. Beth's medical background laid a foundation for her analytical approach to rider position issues.

Beth owns two horses: a promising 2004 mare, Donner Girl ("DG"), and the semiretired 1992 Grand Prix mare, Bluette. She has successfully competed in dressage from Training Level through Grand Prix; has earned her United States Dressage Federation (USDF) bronze, silver, and gold medals; and is a graduate of the USDF "L" judge training program.

When not riding or teaching, Beth can be found in her kitchen exploring new culinary techniques and cuisines, making goat cheese, or joining her husband, David Stutz, for a glass of their Two Barns Vineyard Oregon pinot noir.

Ride in Balance with RiderPilates
exercise DVD

R*ide in Balance with RiderPilates* is for horseback riders of all disciplines and experience levels who want to expand their riding skills. You'll find information and workouts designed to improve your posture, balance and body control in the saddle.

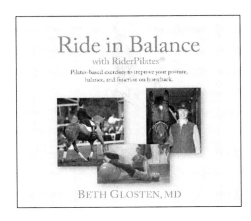

Ride in Balance with RiderPilates includes five chapters:
> Introduction to RiderPilates
> Workout tools — nuts-and-bolts details to start you on the right track
> Basic workout — 34 exercises focusing on body awareness and fundamentals
> Intermediate workout — a more challenging set of 44 exercises
> Preride warm-up — a simple routine you can do anywhere to organize your body before riding

This DVD will help you improve:
> Fitness and body awareness
> Posture and spine alignment
> Stability and balance
> Body control
> Harmony and communication with your horse

**To order *Ride in Balance with RiderPilates*,
go to www.riderpilates.com**

CPSIA information can be obtained at www.ICGtesting.com
Printed in the USA
BVOW060400240912

300911BV00006B/1/P